PANDAS

Reaching out - A natural and homeopathic approach

Grant Bentley

First published in 2016 by Grant Bentley

Copyright © 2016 Grant Bentley

The moral right of the author has been asserted
All rights reserved. No part of this book may be reproduced or transmitted by any person or entity in any form or by any means, electronic or mechanical, including photocopying, recording, scanning or by an information storage and retrieval system, without prior permission in writing from the publisher.

Bentley, Grant
P A N D A S
Reaching out -
A natural and homeopathic approach
Edition: 1st ed.

Produced for Grant Bentley by Louise Bentley
admin@vcch.org
Cover design by Emma Vorozilchak
Printed by
Copyright © 2016 Grant Bentley
All rights reserved.

ISBN-13: 9781536935950
ISBN-10: 1536935956

DEDICATION

As always I dedicate this work to my family and especially to Louise

CONTENTS

Acknowledgments vii
Introduction ix

1	The Syndrome PANDAS	1
2	The Origin of PANDAS	12
3	Two Types of PANDAS	16
4	Convulsive Movements and Tics	23
5	Regression Learning and Personality	28
6	The Action of Stress	35
7	The Nervous and Immune System and Instinct	39
8	The Action of the Survival Instinct	44
9	Sensitivity and Over-reaction	54
10	PANDAS and Food	59
11	Diets and Bacteria	70
12	PANDAS and Exercise	89
13	Obsessions and OCD	99
14	Finding Out About Homeopathy	106
15	Explaining Homeopathy	112
16	Types of Homeopathy	117
17	A New Way to Look at Homeopathy	129
18	E = Energy	133

19	Erroneous Ideas in Homeopathy	136
20	Supportive Parents	140

Find Out More	141
Author Biography	142

ACKNOWLEDGMENTS

Many people have helped me in establishing the ideas that have brought about this book. Samuel Hahnemann's presence looms, as always, over homeopathy. His dedication and continued research to the time of his death has helped me to take his methodology, with my added overlay of facial analysis (HFA), to help many children with PANDAS. The efficacy of homeopathy, along with naturopathic principles, allows for wonderful health outcomes. It is always humbling and amazing to see them unfold.

My thanks also to my colleagues and longtime supporters. In particular, I want to thank all those who have pushed me to keep taking HFA and all it embodies to the world of both practitioners and patients. I would especially like to thank Ellen Kire for her continued dedication to HFA and her encouragement in writing this book.

I would also like to thank all the children and parents who continue to put their trust and hope in me, homeopathy, and in my system. It is a privilege to help with your struggles and then to share in your achievements. A very special thank you goes out to the parents who allowed me to use their children's cases for this book. Names and ages have been changed for anonymity.

Closer to home are my patient and loving family who allow me the time to write and who helped with getting this book to print. The creation of a book is a group effort and my family continue to support me through their interest and their technical, artistic and editorial efforts.

INTRODUCTION

If anyone had asked me over a decade ago what a PANDAS kid is, like most people unacquainted with the syndrome, I probably would have answered that a PANDAS KID is a small black and white bear. However, there is nothing cute or cuddly about the human condition PANDAS.

By training, I am both a naturopath and a homeopath. I have been in full time clinical practice for over twenty years so I am familiar with the many variations of disease presentation. That being said, life still finds ways of surprising you. Over the years, I have treated many syndromes using the same homeopathic principles with success, so it was only a matter of time before I had a very successful outcome with my first PANDAS case. As a result, one happy mother told another struggling mother, and before I knew it, my caseload was filled with predominantly PANDAS cases. Naturally, my proficiency and understanding of the condition grew, and now I am considered an expert in the field.

Many times I have been asked by both homeopaths and parents if there is a book about PANDAS which highlights homeopathy, especially in the way I use it, that is, classical homeopathy with HFA miasmatic diagnosis. As best I am aware there isn't, so this book is my attempt to address PANDAS and homeopathy and answer the fundamental questions of both parents and practitioners.

1

THE SYNDROME PANDAS

PANDAS is an acronym for Pediatric Autoimmune Neuropsychiatric Disorders Associated with Streptococcal infections. But what does that actually mean to the average person? Essentially, a PANDAS kid is a child who displays a range of odd behaviors or a series of emotional and physical changes that are heightened just before, or during, a streptococcal infection.

Streptococcus is an identifying family name for a certain type of bacteria; the type of bacteria that is behind some of our most common conditions, such as the ordinary sore throat. Streptococcus is often the suspect during a sore throat when there are characteristic white patches on the tonsils accompanied with pain and inflammation. Streptococcus or strep, as it's more commonly referred to, is divided into two groups for more accurate identification. Both these groups can cause a varying array of health problems ranging from skin infections, to scarlet fever, to urinary infections, and even pneumonia.

PANDAS as a syndrome was first coined in the nineties after a number of children displaying various motor tics and OCD type behaviors were all found to have the common association of a recent or semi-recent streptococcus infection.

There are a number of ways children are diagnosed as having PANDAS, but essentially PANDAS is any neuropsychiatric disorder that originates after a strep infection. In some cases, a normal happy healthy child after being sick with a sore throat or fever is left with a legacy of causeless fears, motor tics, or OCD (Obsessive Compulsive Disorder) behaviors. However, there is also another group of kids who have a pre-existing neuropsychiatric condition, either officially diagnosed or undiagnosed, and who display symptoms such as OCD behavior, rage, motor tics, or anxieties. These kids fall under the PANDAS category because their already existing condition becomes markedly worse either before or during a strep infection.

One of the first conclusions I observed is that it is not just the streptococcus bacteria by itself that causes such a strong neuropsychiatric response, but the body's own immune response to other stress triggers, including the strep, that brings about the syndrome of symptoms recognized as PANDAS.

Further evidence that PANDAS is an autoimmune neuropsychiatric response rather than an outcome of streptococcal disease alone is observed by the fact that most PANDAS kids will suffer neuropsychiatric exacerbations from a variety of different infections and sensitivities. In fact, a host of other viruses and bacterial infections together with many opportunistic parasites are now being touted as PANDAS triggers.

So for you as the parent of a PANDAS child, the question becomes, what does all this mean? To bring a complex syndrome back to basics, it means PANDAS is a syndrome of behaviors and tics that can often be triggered, or at least exacerbated by, *any* invading infection or parasite. I also want to add that many PANDAS symptoms can also be exacerbated by diet and lifestyle as well as a number of other triggers completely unrelated to strep.

Parents of PANDAS children tell me repeated stories of their child being made markedly worse after eating sugar or gluten, or even when they become stressed by exams or by other school pressures. Many PANDAS kids become noticeably worse after a late night or when they become physically exhausted. Too much sport or too many social activities leaves many PANDAS kids using more energy than they have in reserve and OCD or violent behaviors can result. As a consequence, many PANDAS parents have learned through bitter experience the type of situation that keeps their child in a balanced state as well as the environment that will tip them over the edge.

PANDAS parents will be the first to testify that their household needs to have a routine and be stable. Takeout food, too many late nights, or too many activities that leave their child exhausted, will spell trouble for the week ahead. All factors which lead us to the conclusion that strep alone, cannot possibly be the complete story. The presence of strep is a problem, but we cannot be content to accept that strep alone is the *only* problem and this conclusion changes not only what we think about PANDAS, it also changes how we go about treating it.

Modern chemical medicine is brilliant at killing or destroying. In fact, pain relief and killing invaders is what it does best. So when strep or any other type of bacteria is identified as being the culprit of a syndrome or disease, theoretically, all that needs to be done is to destroy the infection, in this case the strep, and happiness and order will return. However, with PANDAS, this rarely happens. Often, conventional medicine is temporarily effective and its use as a cooperative treatment is not discouraged in my practice. Many times, I have heard accounts of PANDAS kids making remarkable recoveries, even if just temporary, under the persistent use of antibiotics.

Many parents however, do not like the idea of their child taking constant antibiotics because of the changes that take place to the internal flora and good bacteria found in the intestines of their children. Various internal forms of bacteria are vital for breaking down and metabolizing food. Without the correct balance of gut flora (bacteria), a degree of malabsorption and even malnutrition can take place if the condition is severe, and may occur even when the diet is natural and pristine. If the child's diet is anything but clean and healthy then obviously the negative effects of faulty nutrition will be even greater.

Malabsorption of nutrients can create a syndrome with negative consequences that include yeast infections, stubborn painful constipation or chronic diarrhea, fluid retention, muscle loss, failure to thrive, anemia, lethargy, stunted growth, and difficulty concentrating and learning. Many parents of PANDAS kids try to seek out an alternative treatment or at least a therapy they can incorporate alongside their conventional treatment.

A further problem with antibiotic use in the treatment of PANDAS is that often the first course of antibiotics is the most effective, while subsequent courses are less and less so.

Finally, and most importantly, the biggest negative of constant antibiotic use in the treatment of PANDAS is that the only role of the antibiotic is to kill the invading streptococcus bacteria. However, as we have already seen, PANDAS is not only multi-factorial in its triggers, its primary cause is a faulty communication signal within the body itself. In short, this means the biggest contributing factor of PANDAS is not the bacteria that has invaded the patient, but the state of the patient's internal constitution. Following that same train of investigation is the conclusion that the only possible long-term successful treatment plan for anyone diagnosed with PANDAS must be a treatment that not only re-establishes harmonious order within the body, but it must also be a course of treatment whose aim is to strengthen the entire system generally. That plan is beyond the scope of conventional medicine who mostly deny the idea of the constitution, let alone have a medicine to deal with it. Hence, PANDAS parents are forced to seek out alternative practitioners and treatments that help their child on a number of levels. Here is an example of a child I treated and the generalised improvement in their health that followed.

Case 1
Karen - female aged 9 years
Karen's parents first contacted me a couple of years ago when their daughter was nine. At that time, a PANDAS diagnosis was not part of

her presentation, but now I realise Karen's case presented with classic PANDAS symptoms.

Karen's major complaints included OCD thoughts regarding hygiene and germs, anger outbursts, and unreasonable oppositional defiance. She would hit and kick both her mother and her younger sister. Her mother would be at the receiving end of the abuse every time she asked Karen to either clean up her room, or ask her to do anything she did not want to do. Getting her to school was often the worst time of the day, and her tantrums would be out of all proportion to her mother's requests. Frequent claims by Karen that she was going to call the police because of the way her mother was treating her, and often a dogged refusal to get out of the car, were common. Karen's mother, at least a few times a week, would drive home from school in the morning with Karen still sitting, smoldering in the car. Karen's younger sister would also be at the sharp end of her wrath if she happened to win any game the two of them were playing.

Her mother reported that Karen would say the cruelest and most hurtful things, and they were targeted for maximum cutting impact. Karen's mother felt sorry for her youngest daughter because more than anyone else, she was the target of Karen's anger.

On a physical level, Karen always had trouble sleeping. Once she was asleep she was generally okay, but sometimes it would take up to two hours of coaxing, reading, reassuring, and finally threatening, before Karen would shut her eyes. The majority of the time – meaning six nights out of seven – Karen's mother would have to stay with her daughter until she fell asleep, due to her fears of robbers, kidnappers, and ghosts.

Karen was a particularly fussy eater and what she liked and disliked could vary from one week to the next. Some dietary facts were consistent; the first was that she adored meat, and the second that she craved salty food over sweet food, and thirdly she could not eat sugary food or any processed baked goods otherwise her temper would become uncontrollable.

Karen often complained about cramping in her stomach, and although less often, she sometimes felt nauseous and that she might vomit. Sometimes she actually did throw up. The cramping in her stomach was a daily event, while the nausea occurred five days out of the seven. Actual vomiting occurred less often but could be at intervals of once a week.

My general treatment plan always consists of searching for a homeopathic constitutional remedy, combined with discussion about how diet and nutrition could be improved. A conversation about the importance of exercise is another important factor on the road to recovery. Many parents of patients already know much of the information I will tell them regarding diet and exercise, but I always open the discussion as knowledge varies from place to place.

It is also important to point out that the diet and lifestyle discussions I have with parents are delivered on a 'do what you can' basis. Many of the children I treat with PANDAS already have severe oppositional defiance combined with tantrums and sometimes very violent behavior, so I am not going to demand of parents what they should and should not be doing. I just tell them the information they need to hear so they can decide how much of that information is possible to implement in their families lives. However, PANDAS always requires homeopathic remedies. They are a way of calming and balancing the system without the need for constant willpower.

For any reader unacquainted with homeopathy, let me assure you, homeopathy works. I know there is a lot of information out there in the e world, and ninety percent of it is negative towards homeopathy – yes, I have read Wikipedia too – and many times homeopaths themselves do not give their profession as much credibility as it deserves. However, despite all that, homeopathy is highly effective *if* it is used properly.

Two months after beginning her treatment, and with just the one remedy change, Karen's tantrums were reduced. I use a rating system where 10/10 is the worst possible presentation of symptoms and 0/10 means that set of symptoms is gone. Karen's rages and tantrums were 10/10 before the remedy. Karen's mother described her anger two months later as having dropped from 10/10 to 7/10. That is a 30% reduction in two months in her rages. When I checked her sleep pattern, she was still finding it difficult to get to sleep, but there had been a dramatic reduction in the time she spent worrying and talking about ghosts and robbers. Karen's mother estimated that if it took her two hours to fall asleep before taking the remedy, it would now take 30 to 45 minutes on average.

Karen has not been complaining anywhere near as much about her cramping abdomen, and her mother estimated that if it was 10/10 before my treatment, it would be 5/10 now two months later. There had not been any bouts of vomiting and only occasional nausea. The nausea has gone from 10/10 to 3/10 and vomiting from 10/10 to 1/10.

My conclusion was that Karen was doing well on the remedy I chose for her and her mother claimed she was even starting to have more success getting different fruits and vegetables into her diet.

At the next follow up one month later Karen was still on the same remedy and her mother reported that not only had there been a continuous improvement in her rages and fears, she was also getting along with her sister better. Her mother told me how she nearly dropped over with shock when her sister beat Karen at some game they were playing and Karen did not fly into one of her predictable rages. Karen still did not congratulate her sister - homeopathy is a medicine not magic - but as far as social steps forward go, that was a pivotal moment.

One month later after this consultation, I felt Karen was not doing as well – she had stopped progressing and had slipped back a little. So I analyzed her case again and prescribed a new remedy and as before, she began to improve.

A further month after this remedy change, Karen's mother described family life and the house in general as far more relaxed. She said the family was no longer walking on eggshells and she could even ask Karen to clean her room provided she allowed her a certain time frame to comply. Most of the time, the job would be done with a minimum of fuss. It was now a rare day when Karen did not go to school and it also helped that she had made a new friend. Before the remedy, Karen had been much too bossy for any of the other kids to hang around her for too long.

Physically there had been minimal stomach pain. There had been no nausea for quite some time and no vomiting since the second prescription. Karen was even invited to a party where her mother – with trepidation - allowed Karen some party food. She was prepared that the family may end up paying dearly for that indulgence, but it was not the case. In fact, even though she had sugar and cake, Karen remained relatively unaffected that night or the next day. Of course, she could not have kept eating these foods as a regular part of her daily diet, but with the proper treatment, Karen was able to mix with others and not feel singled out.

When I checked with her mother about Karen's general demeanor, her mother said that Karen had always been a more volatile kid generally, and especially by comparison to her laid back sister. However, the fights she was having now, were more like sibling rivalry and in proportion to what a family would normally expect, and very different to the fights that used to occur. The viciousness was gone. Karen's rages and fears, eight months after starting treatment, were assessed by her mother as rating a 2/10. Her abdominal pain was at a low 1/10. Her sleep 4/10, because Karen was still not falling asleep without some reassurance. Her nausea had not returned at all - 0/10.

I still consult with Karen on an occasional basis but I have not needed to treat her for any uncontrollable rages in a long time. More often than not, I treat her for some acute infection or fatigue issues associated with the increasing demands of school. Karen continues to do well in all aspects of her health.

Karen's story is common. It may take a few months for progress to begin and there may be some slipping along the way, but at some point lasting progress will begin for the majority of patients. Patience is required.

PANDAS is more than an acronym for a neuropsychiatric disorder, it also means: **P**atience **A**nd **N**urturing and **D**edication **A**re required for **S**uccess.

For Homeopaths
Without doubt, the foundation of homeopathy is the similimum. Every other principle - posology, potency, intercurrent, and family remedies as well as follow up strategies - are all planets revolving around the sun of the similimum. If you don't have the similimum, you don't have homeopathy. What potency you give is irrelevant if your remedy is wrong. The similimum is everything and the basis of the similimum is the totality of symptoms. I know there is a modern homeopathic ethic of trying to find a single mental symptom or a small group of mental symptoms that represent the spiritual core of the case, if not literally, then at least symbolically, and perhaps this approach is effective in a certain type of case, but it will not be effective in treating PANDAS.

PANDAS is a syndrome that requires a back to basics approach. It is a physical disturbance that requires solid constitutional understanding and accurate prescribing. PANDAS is not an illness for the 'Let's give this a try' homeopath because PANDAS kids have a hypersensitive tendency and will often over-react if the remedy is not a good match. I have developed a way of knowing beforehand whether a certain group of remedies will be right for each patient. This means hypersensitivity is calmed rather than exacerbated.

If you are a homeopathic student, don't get too nervous, remember a similimum is exactly that – similar. Homeopathy does not require that a remedy must be exact. For most patients a few remedies will be required to keep them on their health journey. You are not looking for one perfect remedy that will take them from start to finish. You are looking for the best remedy given the strength and circumstances of the patient at that specific time. As they change or as circumstances change, so too may your remedy choice.

Homeopathic Facial Analysis (HFA) is my secret weapon for success. Every person on the planet has their own predetermined way of dealing with stress or illness. All these varying defensive methods are based on protecting our all- important inner core that houses our vital organs.

When we look at Hering's law – top to bottom, major organs to minor organs, and centre to circumference, it is all just an observation of the body's program of protecting the inner core. The only thing that varies is how we protect it. Different protective strategies are nature's way of not putting all her eggs into the one defense basket.

Some people protect their inner core by throwing disease out to the surface. In this way, even though peripheral areas may suffer such as the skin or the mucous membranes, at least the liver, heart, and kidneys are safe. Other people have inherited a defensive system that is prepared to sacrifice small expendable areas of the body in order to keep their inner core safe. These people have a system that defends itself by capturing and imprisoning any invading virus or bacteria by surrounding it with mucous or inflammation.

When we look at our remedies this trend is the same. Sulphur has a centrifugal action, meaning that it throws what is dangerous out as far as it can away from what is inner and important. While Thuja encapsulates and forms pockets of congestion and inflammation.

Homeopathy works by matching a patient's totality. Not just their presenting signs and symptoms, but the way each patient's immune system tries to fight off disease and re-establish homeostasis.

The way each person defends themselves is the miasm, and the action of the remedy must match that miasm otherwise the patient, especially a PANDAS patient, may react negatively to the remedy. In the HFA system, there are seven miasms and rather than use the traditional disease names (which imply a certain bias towards that disease, which is not true), each group has a color to define it.

The seven groups are yellow, red, blue, orange, purple, green and brown. Everyone belongs to one of these groups. Every remedy belongs to one of these groups. Each miasm/group has corresponding facial features, which is how I work out the miasm for each patient.

HFA uses the concept that a miasm is a defense mechanism. By using an analysis of facial features, I can tell before giving the remedy whether the selected remedy is in harmony with the patient's defense system.

The similimum for Karen's case was found from the following repertorisation -

> MIND; MALICIOUS, spiteful, vindictive (107)
> MIND; STRIKING (74)
> SLEEP; FALLING ASLEEP; late (170)
> GENERALITIES; FOOD and drinks; salt or salty food; desires (59)
> GENERALITIES; FOOD and drinks; meat; desires (52)
> ABDOMEN; PAIN; cramping, griping (461)

Karen's miasmatic classification based on her facial analysis was Tubercular (green group). The remedy that matched both the majority of the repertorised symptoms and her color group (miasm) was Phosphorus. Because PANDAS kids are extremely sensitive, I always choose a lower potency to start, generally 30C. However, because a single dose in a lower potency is not enough to support the case, I repeat the 30C daily.

When Karen needed a change of remedy, I referred back to her original repertorisation because there were no new significant symptoms and the original remedy had been highly effective. Tuberculinum 30C once daily, was my next choice.

2

THE ORIGIN OF PANDAS

What exactly is a neuropsychiatric disorder and why is it associated with a condition like PANDAS? The types of neuropsychiatric problems that present during a PANDAS flare vary enormously and I will discuss them in more detail shortly. As to why they are associated with PANDAS? The truth is no one really knows the physiological pathways that link an immune response to behavioral disorders, let alone why strep or any other infection for that matter should cause a change in neurological or psychological behavior. But the bottom line is they do, or at least they do in susceptible children, and understanding susceptibility is the key.

Many doctors who practice conventional medicine still don't accept that PANDAS is a real phenomenon. Perhaps they think it is all in the imagination of neurotic parents and that the only matter of any psychiatric concern is the mental health of the mother or father. I have met parents who were treated this way.

To me the only questionable aspect of PANDAS is the S at the end. Many of the signs and symptoms displayed by PANDAS kids become exacerbated due to a wide range of circumstances. Too many for me to accept, that the streptococcus bacteria is the major contributing factor, let alone the primary or sole cause. That is not to say that the S for streptococcus is irrelevant, it is not. Parents of susceptible kids will often know there is strep in the school long before the first sniffle or cough is heard by others. Susceptible PANDAS kids can even flare – which means an exacerbation or aggravation of the symptoms – if they even come into contact with a strep carrier. The carrier often does not even know they are a carrier. It is like the Typhoid Mary story, where Mary herself was not sick, but she was a carrier of the infection, meaning she had the infection but not the symptoms. Mary continued mixing with others and infecting them along the way.

However, one thing is for sure. If a PANDAS child is susceptible enough to respond to a strep carrier, it is because their sensitivity generally is out of control. That means they will react to a variety of different triggers ranging from strep to perfumes, to environmental conditions, to numerous foods. Their whole system is way out of balance.

How does a neuropsychiatric disorder present itself? The most common behavioral changes I see in PANDAS kids fall into two categories. The first is OCD behavior, while the second falls under the broad grouping of anger and oppositional defiance.

The most common OCD behaviors include hand washing and a fear of germs or contamination of any kind. This fear of contamination can display itself as an inability or disgust for touching anything that might be perceived as carrying germs, to being incapable of touching a certain item even though consciously the child may recognize that object poses no threat at all.

Hand washing until the skin is raw is often seen. It is also common for a PANDAS child to project their fears onto a particular person. In these cases, the child may know their sister, brother, father, or mother is not actually contaminated, but that knowledge does not help them overcome their fear.

Sometimes the social pressure to overcome their particular fear has the PANDAS child confronting their phobia head on but behind the scenes. Once the confrontation is over an elaborate cleansing ritual will begin in secret. This can range from reciting some sort of chant to a set of behaviors designed to counteract the contamination. Occasionally rituals can take a more serious twist with some PANDAS kids trying to hurt themselves. Often, when asked why they perform their ritual, many will answer that they know what they're doing is illogical and they know their ritual is not really cleansing or protecting them but they are compelled to do it nonetheless, and sometimes to crippling levels. Some bath time rituals include repeated washing, lifting the toilet seat a certain number of times or in a specific way, or even in a certain sequence. This ritualistic behavior can be so difficult that getting a child out of the bathroom and into bed can add an hour or more to the night.

Just as common as OCD is a PANDAS child's need to have a parent close by. Separation anxiety is a common feature and I interpret this as a state of danger they are literally in. PANDAS kids have a real and intense belief that the world is a dangerous and untrustworthy place. This is not part of their own interpretation; I have come to this conclusion myself based on seeing so many kids in this state.

Everything about the PANDAS child shows a nervous system in the grip of fight or flight. Adrenaline surges through their bodies, heightening their sense of hearing and smell, and as their nervous system is on red alert they will see potential danger everywhere. Nearly every aspect of this alarmed state is beyond their conscious control. Thankfully, most of the children I see come from good homes with loving, protective and concerned parents. They have not known violence, except for the violence they themselves cause, and they have not known hardship, often of any kind. Yet they are still in a state of fight or flight.

When I share this observation with parents, especially to a mother, the first thing she does is blame herself. Parents will search in vain for what they might have done, or for what they could do better, to stop this state occurring. For some, it does not matter how much reassurance I give, they still think their actions must be the cause – but that simply is not true. PANDAS kids are born in an impressionable state and as a result they over-react to all sorts of stimuli. Why? I have no idea. Sometimes we just have to deal with what is.

While separation anxiety can be draining on the parent and most often the mother, it usually does not negatively influence the rest of the family. However, OCD rituals can definitely make an impact on everyone, as the fear of breaking a ritual can keep the PANDAS child housebound, resulting in the whole family ending up with cabin fever. However, it is the anger and the oppositional behavior that is often the most exhausting and wounding to everyone.

3

TWO TYPES OF PANDAS

There are two types of PANDAS kids. The first fall into the category of being relatively symptom free most of the time, only to flare up in a major way whenever they are sick or exposed to something they are particularly sensitive to. The second is a group of kids who have disturbing behaviors, most, if not all of the time. They fall into the PANDAS category because their consistent traumatic state is heightened even further when exposed to triggers or when they become sick. This second type have OCD, anger, and fear issues all the time except that they go from 10/10 to 20/10 when their system is thrown out even further.

The first group are a class of kids that can be doing well in school, even being praised for their good work and behavior, then turn into something completely different, throwing the family off guard when they go out of balance. Many times, I have heard the story of how a normally happy and responsive child suddenly turns feral and angry, giving everyone looks that could kill. From being quite balanced, this child begins walking around the house, muttering in whispered tones or singing lines from the same song over and over again. The parents fear for their child's sanity as their PANDAS son or daughter makes them check every corner of the house before sleeping or becomes so angry and defiant that they trash and smash the toys they treasured only forty-eight hours ago. This is a real Jekyll and Hyde scenario. Then, the child gets sick with a fever and all that confusion is explained away. Now everything finally makes sense. Their normally happy child is in the grip of a flare.

Nobody is at his or her best when they are sick, but some PANDAS kids can take this state to a completely new level. Of all the quirky idiosyncrasies during a fever, it is usually the OCD or the anger, or both, that seems to erupt beyond control the most.

PANDAS anger presents at varying levels, just as anger levels vary with everybody else, but with PANDAS, the out of control nature of the anger and sometimes the lack of repentance afterwards is what differentiates these outbursts from what is generally considered normal. Most parents have a reasonably good idea of normalcy regarding emotions. As with Karen's mother in the first case history I presented, she knew the difference between sibling rivalry and expected preteen behavior, and that it was different for Karen during a PANDAS flare.

Case 2
Edward – male aged 13 years.
Edward's mother described her son as having been quirky and a little on the edge since he was a young boy. He would scream if he saw a bee or a wasp and almost jump into his mother's arms if a dog was anywhere nearby. He would need the same bedtime reassurances every night otherwise he would have nightmares. As a very young child Edward was happy go lucky and exceptionally bright for his age. His vocabulary at four was as good as his older sisters at seven. At the age of four, Edward had a series of vaccinations. It was straight after this, according to his mother, that Edward stopped speaking for nearly a year. When his speech finally did return, it was far more limited and far less expressive than it had been before.

By the age of seven, Edward was mostly back on track and progressing nicely and normally again, when his father was involved in a near fatal car accident that left him hospitalized for eight months.

His father's near death accident left Edward shocked and shaken and that is when even deeper fears began.

On questioning, his mother admitted that Edward had always been on the nervous side and that he needed more reassurance than any of her other children. However, the anxiety she was used to experiencing from Edward was entirely different to the fears she was beginning to witness. She had been used to a 'tell me everything is going to be alright,' type of anxiety from her son, but now Edward was too scared to come out of his room. He was too scared to have a shower in case someone had 'accidently' put gas into the pipes. He had also developed an extreme type of hypochondria and constantly stayed in bed with his computer researching every ache and pain he experienced.

As well as fears, Edward also started developing a number of crippling OCD behaviors. He started walking in two directions only – straight ahead and to his right. If he needed to turn left for any reason, Edward would have to walk in a wide circling loop in order to get to where he wanted to go. However, what became of extreme concern was Edward's new tendency toward rage and violence.

Edward had always been a bright boy, but he had become an unpredictable and violent teen, paranoid in the extreme, self-loathing, yet full of self-grandeur at the same time. During his periods of loathing, he would cut and hit himself and then scream out in pain at what he had done. If his parents came into the room, the very sight of them, especially his mother, would send Edward into a rage because he did not want to be looked at. Before working with me, Edward's mother had contacted numerous psychiatrists. She had also been to psychologists, social workers, and healers of every description. He had been hospitalized twice - once after a serious suicide attempt – and another, when the police had been called due to a violent attack on his mother, where he bashed her in the head after she came in to his room without warning to collect his dinner dishes. After this, they both decided on a routine where she would ring a bell outside his room which would give him five minutes notice before she was about to enter.

Edward could not go to the toilet because he was too scared to leave his room. At the same time, he believed that God had personally chosen him for some great and important work that was to occur in the near future.

Edward did not go to school and yet despite his torturing and tormenting thoughts, remained a bright intelligent teenager. One part of Edward knew he could not conquer his fears, but at the same time, he was lonely and missed the company of others his own age. He talked a little on social chat from time to time, but in the end had given up because he had no common shared experiences to talk about.

Edward was allergic to a range of foods, especially gluten based foods, which his mother assured me made his mental symptoms much worse. The household environment was stable but distant. Edward's mother described her marriage as a contract to stay calm rather than anything loving and supportive. Edward's father believed his son needed to be committed either fully or at least for more extended periods than the brief respite they received. Edward's mother said this had caused a huge rift in their marriage, as she did not want him to be sent away and she was prepared to sacrifice everything to look after her son.

Her two other children had their own problems. Edward's younger brother also suffered from fears and experienced tics, although nowhere near to the same degree. Edward's older sister seemed stable but both were highly resentful of the time Edward demanded of their mother. Edward's father spent a lot of time with both his daughter and his youngest son in an attempt to make up for the shortfall.

The family had first contacted me to help them with their youngest son Richard, not Edward. Thankfully, I am happy to say Richard did very well after treatment.

When Edward was first booked in to see me (via Skype, not in my clinic), I was not sure how much I could achieve. For reasons I will go into later in the book, the more a person is consistently disturbed in their behavior, the less chance of recovery and improvement there is. I know that sounds blunt but that is what I have seen.

When I first started treating Edward's younger brother Richard, he had symptoms of hypochondria and separation anxiety. He also had some facial tics where he would blink very rapidly and stretch his neck to one side. However, there was a very big difference between Richard and Edward. Richard's symptoms would be most apparent before a sore throat or when he was exhausted, but Edward was caught in the grip of his symptoms 24/7. There was never any relief for Edward and that unfortunately means treatment will take a much slower pathway.

After six months of treating the younger brother Richard, he was easily able to leave his mother to go off and play with his friends. He began to attend school more than being at home. This was a huge difference by comparison to how he was prior to treatment, where he was often home in bed with a pain somewhere.

After eight months of treatment, Richard had become a valuable member of a local sporting team and even stayed over at friend's houses when asked. He was no longer even close to being a hypochondriac. Edward's progress however was a different story.

After a year of working with Edward, while there had been some gains, they were not as great as his younger brother Richard's improvements. Edward was not spending all his time in his room in the dark as when I first started working with him, in fact he was leaving his room quite frequently. Although he had not left the house yet, there was hope that time would come. He was showering and eating well and even doing some homework. Edward was still feeling the pressure of the greatness he perceived was coming in the future, but he was no longer violently aggressive and he had not hit his mother since the third remedy of treatment. He was no longer walking in wide loops to get where he wanted to go and he had even rung his cousin on the phone on occasions. On good days, Edward would occasionally play an electronic game with his sister or brother.

His improvements were not overall consistent, but they were enough to put light into his mother's heart.

Edward's case is still a work in progress, so I guess the question you the reader may have is why did I choose to put such a case into a book instead of selecting a miracle cure? The answer is because this gradual and less distinctive response is the most common response for PANDAS kids who fall into group two like Edward. Sometimes miracles do occur with these severely damaged children, but by their very nature they are rare.

When treating kids with PANDAS, it is important to offer hope but also to be realistic with expectations. Having a boy like Edward able to leave his room is a big step indeed. Anyone who doubts that breaking an obsession like this is a big step forward has never had an OCD child. The fact that Edward will shower most days and will even go to the toilet on his own is a huge improvement compared to when he first presented for treatment. How much further Edward can go is anybody's guess. Every patient who sees a practitioner wants to believe his or her practitioner knows exactly what will happen every step of the way, but unfortunately that is just not true. People are all individual and to what extent a patient will or will not respond is often unknown beforehand. I often have a reasonably good idea based on prior experience, but sometimes you just don't know and you have to be an observer and watch and guide as the case unfolds.

For Homeopaths
The rubrics I chose for Edward's case were -

> MIND; FEAR; happen; something will (98)
> MIND; HYPOCHONDRIASIS (136)
> MIND; RAGE, fury (139)
> MIND; LOOKED at; cannot bear to be (27)
> MIND; VIOLENCE, vehemence (124)

His miasm based on facial analysis took me three attempts to work out. Facial analysis with teens who are both damaged and non-compliant can make the process take longer than I would otherwise like, but with perseverance and the help of parents, I can usually work out this first step and then choose remedies that will resonate at a deeper level. Once I placed him in the orange color group (Syco-psoric miasm) he began to show a response. The third remedy selected, based on rubrics and color grouping, was Nux Vomica 30C once daily.

Color grouping is another classification for the miasm. There is more information about HFA and miasms in the homeopathy section and at the end of the book.

4

CONVULSIVE MOVEMENTS AND TICS

Another part of the neuropsychiatric picture is the many convulsive movements, grimaces and tics that PANDAS patients suffer. These play a large part of the syndrome of PANDAS and they are the symptoms that put the neuro into neuropsychiatric.

Tic presentations in PANDAS can be divided into two types. These types are not exclusive, which means having one type does not prevent you from developing the other, in fact, many PANDAS kids have both. The first type of tic is a physical tic, often referred to as a motor tic. Within this category, another further classification can be made by dividing motor tics into the terms simple and complex.

A motor tic is an involuntary motion or jerking of a muscle. If this involuntary motion affects only one area of the body, such as the raising up of one side of the mouth, then that tic is a simple tic. More commonly seen with PANDAS children is a series of movements. For example, the child may raise one side of the mouth, followed by a set of rapid eye blinking, then a roll of the neck. That series of tics is regarded as a complex motor tic rather than the one symptom single tic.

The second category of tics is the vocal tic and this is especially common in PANDAS, particularly with younger children. Like motor tics, vocal tics involve the same numerous repetitive occurrences, except a word or a sound is repeated rather than a movement of the body or face.

As part of the PANDAS syndrome most of these tics, both vocal and motor, are involuntary. There is another term that is often applied to tics; the term unvoluntary. Involuntary tics can often be controlled or suppressed by a sheer act of will. Unvoluntary tics by contrast, cannot be controlled by any act of will. In the old days where harsher terminology was common to describe mental pathology, unvoluntary motions or tics would be associated with mentally retarded people. Uncontrollable swaying or rocking would be one example.

PANDAS tics are mostly of the controlled variety. Parents describe their child as a devil inside the home but an angel outside. Often this is because outside the home the child engages all their willpower to keep their tics under control so their peers will not see them. However, as anyone who has ever been on a diet or an exercise program, or even wanting to push through to achieve something within a certain time period, will tell you, willpower takes a lot of energy. After a day of suppressing their tics, or at least being crafty enough to invent some strategies so their tics pass unnoticed, the PANDAS child often returns home drained and needing to let go completely. Suppressing symptoms through willpower often applies to negative behavioral problems and this is where some PANDAS kids get their Jekyll and Hyde reputation.

I have had many confused mothers telling me how their child's teacher would be shocked to learn that their child is so badly behaved at home, let alone struggling with tics.

This involuntary rather than unvoluntary condition has also led to countless family disagreements, often with the father arguing with the mother that their child is only behaving this way because YOU are enabling them and allowing them to get away with it. The mother's response is often an attempt to reassure the father that she is NOT to blame and that she is trying everything she can, including tenderness, as well as discipline, but the child keeps breaking down.

For many PANDAS kids, home is a place of release and where they can finally let the cat out of the bag so to speak. That does not make life any easier for those in the home, but at least understanding why is a start.

The variety of tics PANDAS kids can suffer from is numerous, but the most common area seems to be the head and face, however this is not exclusive. Facial tics range from eye squinting, to scrunching up and twitching the nose, to going cross-eyed, or rolling the neck and head.

Other common areas include hand flapping or restless legs. Often the hand-flapping tic strikes fear into a parent because of its autistic implications. However, hand flapping alone does not indicate autism.

In many ways PANDAS can seem to imitate autism, especially when there are vocal tics involved because the vocal tic can seem like a form of stimming (self-stimulatory behavior) that is common with autistic children. The regressive behavior of PANDAS can also seem to imitate autism, but with PANDAS the onset is sudden, and after a flare, the child returns to their normal state. True autism is much harder to treat than PANDAS. They are two completely different conditions even though on the surface they share some cross over symptoms.

Tics are a common accompaniment to the PANDAS syndrome and although children with autism can have tics, it is not a major piece in the identification puzzle like it is with PANDAS.

Tics are linked to fear and anxiety, which is why they are so common in PANDAS. The good news is that I have treated a large number of PANDAS kids and many have had their tics dramatically reduce in severity and frequency, while for others their tics have gone completely.

When the tics are first noticed, some parents become very upset watching their child endure these involuntary motions, and often what makes them most upset is why their child just doesn't stop. 'Just tell yourself not to do it.' However, it is not that easy. Sure, it can be done for a while, with willpower and best behavior, but a tic is far more than a habit.

A tic is an urge. Smoking for example is a habit, whereas breathing and blinking are compulsive necessities, and a tic has that same compulsive demand. If you hold your breath for as long as you can, your body begins to tighten and contract, and an overall sense of stress sets in. Then, as you finally release your breath and quickly inhale a new batch of fresh air, your body relaxes and you are happy again. This is what it is like to have a tic. A tic is a demanding urge that will just not go away. Instead, it continues to build until even more stress and discomfort sets in. The physical expression of the tic, such as head rolling or the eyes being squeezed together, creates the same sense of relief as the release of the held breath followed by the inspiration of new fresh air.

While tics seem to be more common in males than females, a number of female PANDAS sufferers also experience tics. Sometimes these tics are mainly present during conscious waking hours. When the child falls asleep, their body, or more specifically their nervous system, gives them some peace and allows them to relax and refresh. However, some kids are not so fortunate. For some PANDAS kids, the tics remain constant through the night even while they sleep. Parents report how their child's body will suddenly jump or jerk, or they may toss and turn restlessly throughout the night. Often, these kids will also have dark circles under the eyes and react strongly to stimulants like sugar.

All these symptoms point to the conclusion that they are enduring a heavy drain on their adrenal glands and that their body is burning energy it does not really have.

Using adrenalin as an energy source for the body is not uncommon for this type of PANDAS patient. The adrenal glands sit right above the kidneys, and any long-term demand on the adrenals forces the glands to steal energy from the larger energy reservoir of the kidneys. Once a child reaches this stage, a number of kidney-bladder symptoms can start presenting themselves. A constant urge to urinate becomes a common accompaniment to a PANDAS flare. This stage can also exhibit itself in symptoms such as a loss of bladder control, either partial or complete. By partial I mean, and this is mainly with boys, that their – how can I put this delicately – their aim becomes poor. Many times, I have heard the complaint that the bathroom has urine everywhere except in the bowl itself. Sometimes it can seem as if someone has gone into the bathroom with a high-pressure hose turned on full and left it swiveling and thrashing all over the place. What else could explain why there is urine on the floor and on the walls, in fact urine everywhere except in the toilet?

For PANDAS girls, being a part-time firefighter is not anatomically possible, but adrenal exhaustion can leave them prone to bladder infections during or after a flare. Generally, these infections are mild, and most often tests reveal nothing untoward in the urine, such as a bacterial infection, even though the signs and symptoms might suggest otherwise. Usually an increase in the frequency to urinate is seen, sometimes accompanied by a mild tingling or burning.

But it is the vocal tics that panic parents the most, especially after the first PANDAS flare occurs. Seeing their child, who seemed so normal only a short time ago, walking around the house whispering to themselves, or repeating the same phrases over and over, is highly disconcerting and can have the new comer to PANDAS questioning their child's sanity.

5

REGRESSION LEARNING AND PERSONALITY

There is nothing backward about the PANDAS child. During a flare, there can be a mental and emotional regression, but thankfully this regression is, in most cases, temporary. By mental regression, I mean that learning anything new can become extremely difficult and in many cases impossible. Handwriting can regress backwards from an age appropriate level, as can other fine motor skills like catching, hitting, or throwing a ball. The willingness to learn can become non-existent, but even though the child cannot be bothered with any new information, they thankfully do not unlearn what they already know. After the flare, most children go back to their old selves, their hand writing returns to the level it was before the PANDAS, and their interest in the outside world increases as the grip of their OCD lessens.

Many PANDAS kids however, do not start from a balanced or a 'normal' place. What is normal for them might not be exactly what the average person may consider normal. In the previous paragraph, I am talking about a child who is balanced in every respect until a PANDAS flare up begins. However, I have to tell you that most PANDAS kids do not fall into this category. Most are best described as either anxious, quirky, a little on edge, or that they have their little habits. Generally, these habits are not debilitating, and more often than not, no one outside of the immediate family even knows they exist. They are what used to be referred to as minor idiosyncrasies; those unpredictable desires or habits that go to mold the uniqueness of character.

Okay, so not everybody has these traits, but if they are not debilitating and they do not stop the child from mixing or doing anything they want to do, then it's a character trait that is just…well, them. Provided they can socialize well with friends, play their part on their local sporting team, learn the subjects that are important to them, and at least pick up enough information to pass a test on the subjects that aren't of interest, who cares if they have their unique ways. And by the way, boys not paying attention or even trying with any subject they aren't interested in, yet focusing for hours on topics they love, is not PANDAS or autism or any other sort of label. That is a boy being a boy. And one more addition, remedies do not make teenagers clean their rooms!

Understanding the starting point of a PANDAS constitution is vital for predicting how far any treatment can go. Remedies, diet, exercise, and supplements, are vital for restoring health, but there comes a time when everyone has to accept what part is the child's inherent personality and what part are the signs and symptoms that show their system is under stress and out of balance. Signs and symptoms of an out of balance state, I can do something about, but changing a person's personality is impossible.

It is important to understand what is achievable. If a child was happy, active, and able to learn before their PANDAS flare, then it is definitely possible to bring them back to that point. If a child was always the anxious type, but then after PANDAS they became housebound and terrified, and then their tics started, returning them to a tic free state and able to socialize with friends again, would be achievable. However, this second child will probably still be a bit of a worrier even after the treatment has been completed, because that is the natural state of their personality.

If a child is autistic and the signs became obvious right from their early development, I might be able to help in some of the allied traits or symptoms that can accompany autism, but I can rarely remove the autism. I say rarely because I did have a case where a young boy with autism was brought to me to help with his repeated coughs and colds. He was congested all the time and he did not talk but would grunt and point. He was considered hyperactive and had the classic autistic behaviors of lining up toys. Green mucus was always dripping from his nose and regular bouts of bronchitis during winter were common.

After finding the right remedy for this boy, his congestion started clearing dramatically but not only that, he started talking. Previously he had never spoken but would just point, grunt or make noises. He would not look his father in the eye when his father tried to talk with him. He never smiled at anyone or acknowledged their presence. He was totally removed and totally self-contained. Because the remedy I had him on was doing such a good job at keeping him well – he had gone all winter without any bronchitis, which was the first winter ever – plus he had spoken a few words in a sentence, I decided to keep the remedy going to see where it would take him.

I saw this boy over a few months and then after a year. I also had a phone follow up after three years. This little boy who had been in a special needs school was about to start in a new public school because his original diagnosis of a 'special needs' child had been reversed. Now not only could he connect with others, he would sit up and smile as he read books with his dad before going to sleep. He had also just joined a football team. He and his father moved interstate after that and I never heard what happened longer term, but I was so amazed by what I had witnessed, that I wrote the case up in a professional journal. A few parents with severely autistic children came to see me after that case in the hope I could replicate that same result for them. Sadly, I have never been able to achieve that same result, although I have been able to help in other ways. For example, if an autistic child was violent or they were having trouble with congestion or digestion, I have been able to help in those areas significantly, but this little boy has been the only case I can think of to have an autism diagnosis completely reversed.

So what exactly can be achieved in the treatment of PANDAS? The answer is quite a lot, but it depends on the severity of the case and also the state of the child's constitution before the PANDAS flare.

Case 3
Jimmy – male aged 10 years.
A few years ago, I received a request for an international booking for a young boy named Jimmy. A large proportion of my clients are from overseas, in particular the USA. In fact, US patients have become such a large portion of my daily practice, that I now treat more US kids and adults than Australians. Jimmy lived in the North West of the United States and while he had PANDAS flares all year round, they were particularly bad in the spring and in the autumn/fall because of the molds that grow on the wet and rotting leaves. Jimmy's allergies would weaken his body due to his constant sneezing, sleep loss, and the energy it took to create a constant immune response. Spending each day in a continual immunological battle is exhausting to the body. Every spring and every autumn/fall, Jimmy would sneeze and itch until finally his PANDAS would flare. Once at this stage, Jimmy would become aggressive towards his family and sometimes he would even hit and kick in frustration if his allergies were bad enough. He would start to tic by pulling faces, squinting, and raising his eyebrows up and down. He would also move his head in a manner that looked like he was trying to touch his right shoulder with his chin.

If the allergies were really bad, his OCD would also kick in, and then he would be compelled to touch anything brown or orange in color, or anything smooth to his fingers. He had to touch these objects in a tapping motion, with each series of touches consisting of blocks of seven taps. This meant that in the kitchen for example, where the dining table was made of polished wood, he was compelled to enter the room and go straight to the table – tap tap tap tap tap tap tap – seven taps make one touch, and every brown, orange, or smooth object had to be touched twice.

Jimmy would plead to his mother how much he hated his tics and his OCD. He would tell her that he felt like a freak and that he wanted more than anything to stop, but he couldn't. He would lie awake worrying at night and crying himself to sleep. His mother too would be crying in the next room, but Jimmy never knew that. His father first contacted me, which is very unusual because normally mothers make the first contact. The mother is usually the person most prepared to give alternate health options a try, while the father often states that he knows for a fact that all this alternate stuff is rubbish. How these guys 'know for a fact', that alternative therapies are rubbish, when they really know nothing about them is beyond me, but it is a very common occurrence. Perhaps men are more persuaded by some of the anti-alternative 'information' that springs up on the internet whenever a viable scientific study shows that alternative treatments have something to offer?

This time however, it was different, as a very concerned father and husband contacted me as to what could be done.

After finally getting onto a good remedy for Jimmy, which initially took me a few consultations to find, he began to respond in a positive way. The first response was with his allergies. Every night Jimmy had needed to be nebulized in order to be able to breathe easily enough to sleep. The nebulizer was the first thing to go. By go, I mean, not used unless it had to be. I do not mean thrown away; that should never be done in case an emergency occurs. The need to nebulize diminished rapidly and what had been a nightly routine, evaporated into a once every second night, to once every third or fourth, to once a week, to if required. The gurgling sound of the lodged congestion in Jimmy's throat and chest also began to break up and clear. His sleeping improved and over the course of the next three months, his tics virtually disappeared. Most importantly for Jimmy, who didn't care so much about the tics, and even less about the allergies, was that his OCD compulsion to touch was markedly better two months after finding the right remedy, and gone by the third month.

Over the summer, Jimmy remained well, but summer was always his best time anyway, so his health was expected to be good. Then came the dreaded change from summer to autumn/fall, and while there were a few times when his allergies would recommence at a low level, Jimmy essentially got through the season relatively symptom free. I say relatively because there were a few times when I had to readjust the frequency of his dose. His tics returned for a few days in a row, along with his OCD touching. If before they were 10/10 in their severity, this time they were both no more than 3/10 – enough to let everybody know that they were still lurking in the background, but not enough to interrupt the family's routine, and certainly not enough to make Jimmy start worrying again. Within a few days of beginning, his tics and OCD stopped again.

I still keep in semi-regular contact with Jimmy, especially over the spring and autumn, and he continues to do well. No one else would have any idea that he had experienced some severe PANDAS flares.

One of the main things I noticed in Jimmy's case was the absence of any streptococcus infection. He had tested positive when the first flare sent Jimmy and his mother to the doctors, but most of the time Jimmy's PANDAS flares were caused by an over burdening of his system, due to his severe response to seasonal allergies. Most of his PANDAS flares had no association with strep at all.

The allergies Jimmy suffered from were more than enough to drain his system of whatever energy he had left. In many ways, energy levels are a much better way of understanding the fluctuations of PANDAS, instead of looking for an infection that may or may not be the base line cause.

For Homeopaths

The symptoms I chose for Jimmy's repertorisation were -

NOSE; CORYZA; annual, hay fever (127)
MIND; GESTURES, makes (142)
RESPIRATION; ASTHMATIC; night (49)
GENERALITIES; TOUCH; agg. (200)

The rubric 'Gestures' was used to describe the many facial tics that were occurring. The rubric 'Touch aggravates' under the generals was chosen instead of the mind rubric 'Impelled to touch things' because this latter rubric has only 10 remedies, whereas the rubric 'Touch aggravates' has 200. I do not agree with small rubric selection especially in the beginning of a case, because I want to keep my remedy options open. Even though this repertorisation contains rubrics of a moderate to large size, there were still only 16 remedies that covered all of the rubrics. Jimmy's facial analysis showed he belonged to the red color group (sycotic miasm) which narrowed the 16 available remedy choices down to 3.

The reason it took me a number of attempts before I got the right remedy was because the photos originally taken of Jimmy by his parents, were very poor in quality, making his facial analysis difficult. I originally placed Jimmy in an incorrect color group which is why none of the first remedies I chose for him worked very well. This also highlights how vital it is for parents to follow the photo taking instructions.

Once I had examined the new set of photos I requested, it became obvious why Jimmy wasn't responding. Once I knew definitely he was red (this is the type of defense system that protects the core by building a barrier around bacteria and any other danger) all I had to do was go back to my repertorisation and select the highest ranking red remedy (one that shares the same defensive action as the patient). The red remedy I chose was Antimonium Tartaricum 30C, one dose daily.

6

THE ACTION OF STRESS

It is better to think of PANDAS as a syndrome of predictable symptoms that rise to the surface whenever the body is under stress. That being said, it becomes important to discuss exactly what stress is. Perhaps one of the best ways to start is by defining what stress is not. For one thing, stress is not just an emotional response. People generally think of stress as an emotional reaction and a state of tension. Being stressed and being upset are regarded as two interchangeable terms, but this is not only the case. Stress is anything and everything that can upset the equilibrium of the body. Therefore, stress can come from too much junk food, too much emotional trauma, too much exercise, or too little exercise. Stress can result from too many late nights, too heavy a workload or, as can be seen in Jimmy's case, by repeated acute infections and/or allergies.

Imagine that inside your child's body is a set of old world scales with a small measuring plate either side of the gauge. On one side of the scales is the appropriate energy level for the child; on the other side of the scales is the syndrome of symptoms that make up your child's PANDAS condition. Let us pretend at this moment that both sides are equally balanced. But what would happen if the scale that holds your child's energy up were to drop down? That is right, the other side of the scale, the plate that holds your child's PANDAS signs and symptoms, would go up. It is as simple and as complicated as that.

Simple because through a model of this type, we begin to understand that stress is classified as anything that disturbs an individual's harmonious level of energy balance. Complicated, because that could mean anything.

Knowing your child is stressed is easy because they have the PANDAS signs and symptoms to tell you. What caused that stress is the unknown factor, which is why I encourage my patients to start keeping a simple health diary about their child. The diary does not have to be extensive, just a note of whether their child had a good or bad day, when it comes to their symptoms. If they had a bad day, make a note of what was going on around them. Was it a Monday after a busy weekend, or was it after a party, or after an outing where more processed foods were eaten? When you look back at their diary, is there any pattern emerging? For example, have you noticed that a bad day seems to occur every Friday or every Wednesday? Even if you cannot pinpoint why, it still tells us that there is an element of periodicity in your child's PANDAS case. If they seem to have a major flare every month instead of every week, take note of what is happening around them. Is it roughly the same time every month? If so, your child's PANDAS symptoms may be linked to the phases of the moon. Rubbish, you think. Then think again, because many parents after being instructed to keep a health diary, have discovered exactly what I am saying is true. That is how I know.

Why would the moon have any impact of PANDAS? Well it probably doesn't directly, but indirectly its effect can be strong. A weakened system, for whatever reason, can fall prey to a host of opportunistic bacteria, worms, and parasites, and it's probably these things, and not the PANDAS itself, that are reacting to the cycles of the moon. Certain types of worms and bacteria are known to have their breeding cycles linked to the phases of the moon.

When a carnivorous hunting animal goes in search of its prey, it rarely strikes at the strongest and healthiest victim. Usually, a hunter prefers to target the old, the weak, or the one lagging behind because they will not put up too much resistance. When lions or dogs attack a larger grazing animal, they always go for the most defenseless. They may be hungry, but they have no intention of putting themselves in harm's way by attacking an animal that might fight back and hurt them.

Human beings are just the same. The healthier we are, the greater chance we have of warding off any invading opportunistic infection. If our immune system is operating well, and it can search out, destroy, and recognize non-self from self, then we can get on with life with a minimum of fuss. However, when our immune system is struggling to keep up with demands, suddenly we start to feel sick more often. Even if we don't get the flu or some other type of infection, we can often feel as if we are always on the verge of getting one, even to the point of feeling achy, cold, and feverish, yet nothing ever seems to eventuate.

I can always tell when a child's immune system is working too hard, or is under par, because one sickness seems to roll into another. Instead of having one or two colds a year, a child with an under-functioning immune system has one cold that seems to run into the next. Sometimes, in children who have this condition, nature can be kind and give them a week or two break before another cold or another fever takes its grip again. Others however are not so lucky, and parents of these children describe their child as only getting two colds a year, the first one lasting from December to June, while the second goes from September to late November. If there is a child like this in the family, more often than not it will be your PANDAS child.

A child's nervous system can behave in exactly the same way as the immune system, in fact, one is integrally linked to the other. A nervous system that runs on high, without any down time or relaxation, drives the rest of the body to the point of exhaustion – and this is common with PANDAS kids. Most are already more anxious by nature but that does not mean they are always in a panic. Even when they are not in a flare, the PANDAS child is often the one who needs that little extra reassurance. They are often the child, even in good times, to need someone close – just in case. They are also the one you need to watch more when it comes to diet and adverse reactions. Which leads us back to the necessity of a diary.

Even if your PANDAS child is not anxious by nature, they will often be the child that is the most sensitive to their surroundings, the most reactive, and on a positive note, often the sharpest and the most observant.

Reaction and sensitivity go hand in hand; you cannot have one without the other. So while your PANDAS child may be the most affectionate or the wisest of all your children, they will also be the most reactive. This is why many PANDAS children suffer from allergies and various food intolerances.

7

THE NERVOUS AND IMMUNE SYSTEM AND INSTINCT

Why does someone so anxious or sensitive also have so many immunological problems? When the nervous system is on red alert - as it is with most PANDAS kids - the whole system is operating at a frenzied level and just like when you run around in a fluster, two things generally happen; the first is you make mistakes, and the second is you become tired.

PANDAS kids, for whatever reason, have a highly strung nervous system that they were born with, or they have been put into a state of red alert through an event or a series of events. I spoke about this earlier when I was talking about fight or flight but what does that actually mean?

Fight or flight is an inbuilt programmed response to danger. It is instinctive, which means you do not have to think about it, but that has both its upside and its downside.

Our body does most important daily activities without the need of our awareness or consent. We can overrule these instincts of course and jump in front of a car if we really want to, but thankfully, most of us rarely reach that state. For the most part, each and every day, there are two different lives going on both around us and inside of us and there are two driving forces that control these two worlds; the first is consciousness, and the second is instinct.

Consciousness is best described as a state of awareness. It is not how smart we are, because that is a byproduct of genetics and drive. Awareness, without getting too out there and spiritual, is the state or the ability to observe.

To understand awareness fully you need to accept that there are two different aspects to this puzzle. One is the observer and the other is the observed. The observed is usually some sort of object, or it could be another person, or it could be oneself. That is how we know awareness is separate to logic, emotions, intelligence, or feelings, because we can observe them all.

However, you can only observe what is separate to you. You can observe a dog because you are separate from that dog. You can observe your thoughts because you are separate from your thoughts, but you cannot observe your awareness or yourself because you are your awareness. Got it? Good, because there will be a pass or fail exam on this at the end of this chapter. Okay, I admit that is not true, but consciousness or awareness, whichever term you understand the most, is the prime driving force behind most of the thoughtful part of our life. It is that part of us that lets us know we are alive and appreciating the impressions our senses are bringing in. It is that part of us we often refer to when we talk in terms of 'I'. I like this or I want to do that. I have an ambition to… or I love it when… It is the 'I' that loves music. The ears may be the sensory medium that brings music to your attention, but your ears do not discriminate or love anything they hear, they just trap certain amplitudes and frequencies so your brain can then decipher them. YOU hear music; your ears just capture sound.

I know I have taken you a long way from the signs and symptoms of PANDAS but there is a point to this, and to make this point clear, I need to discuss the next dominating force in human life and that is the force of instinct.

Instinct is the complete opposite of conscious awareness, however its role is just as dominant, in fact, during periods of stress, instinct is even more dominant than awareness.

Every organic creature, to a lesser or greater extent, has instinct. The seed does not think about bursting and sprouting into a tree, it just does it. Worms and snails do not think about recoiling when you touch them, they just react. They don't think about what is touching them or whether what is touching them means them harm or not, the snail just recoils into its shell and after an allotted time has passed, it ventures out once again. The point is, when I say that all organic creatures have an instinct as a dominant force, organic creatures also means you and your PANDAS child.

The difference between human beings and other animals is that human beings are not just instinct. We have the ability to be conscious of who we are, and we have a complex proprioception network as well as an awareness of time and space that go far beyond anything else on the planet. This is why we can plan for tomorrow – because we understand the concept of tomorrow. Your pet dog has no comprehension of time or that there is a tomorrow.

You may have had your beloved pet dog for many years and how many times has your dog missed out on its meal? Most likely never. Does the fact that you are going to feed it tomorrow and the next day and the day after that stop it from gulping down its food as quickly as it can? Have you ever known your dog to slow down, take a mouthful of food, then savor its flavor like some taste connoisseur on Master Chef? No, never, not once in all the time you have fed your pet has your dog ever bothered to slow down and enjoy its meal. That is instinct in action. A program that dominates and controls every action of every animal, so it does not have to stop and think about what it is doing because it does not have the natural capacity to do so.

Instinct is instilled into every living creature so it does not have to think about all the things it has to do just to survive. It is nature's way of helping us. We go about our daily lives doing the things we either want or have to do. We do not stop to think about the best way to digest that apple we just ate, or the pasta we had for lunch. We may think afterwards that we have to stop eating so much pasta for lunch, but that is a different issue.

We never think about what we have to do to digest and assimilate a meal nor do we consider how best to distribute its nutrients, mainly because we don't have the faintest clue of how to do it, it is just way too complicated, so all these actions are done for us automatically. You can focus on your breathing while doing yoga or meditation but you do not have to. You do not know how to make your red blood cells take up oxygen for transport around your body, much less how to control your white cells for the job of immunity. In fact, we do not know how to do many of the processes that keeps us alive every day. All of these things come under the category of instinct. Awareness may control your thoughts but instinct controls your body. However, there are also times when instinct takes control of our thoughts and consciousness is relegated to the background. This is when we go into fight or flight.

The link between consciousness/awareness and instinct applies to PANDAS. PANDAS kids seem to be in a constant state of fight or flight and as a result, they see the world through the eyes of danger, rather than a place full of adventure and exploration. This is not to say that conscious awareness does not exist for PANDAS kids. Even during times of danger our awareness is still present, but awareness is not the captain of the ship; it is more like the first mate. In fact, most of the time when parents share with me that their child had a good day or a good week, the 'good' is defined by how aware their child has been and how much their survival instinct has been under control and operating within acceptable limits.

When conscious awareness is captain of the ship, children are able to explore and venture out, meet other people and discover new boundaries that they would not normally feel safe enough to do. When the survival instinct is captain, all it cares about is safety and protection, and the best way of achieving protection is to always have a more competent person close by. Which is why separation anxiety is so common with the PANDAS child.

Another way of keeping their own environment safe is by keeping their surroundings small and unchanging. This is why your PANDAS child is such a fussy eater and it is why he or she gets so upset and rages against anything that takes them out of their comfort zone. You will see them wanting to have one or two closer friends rather than hanging out with a larger group. This constant sense of threat and need for security will not let the PANDAS child experience peace until their survival instinct is reassured that they are out of danger. Only then will consciousness return to its dominant place.

The other important aspect to remember about the survival instinct is that it controls the body. So when the survival instinct is in a state of alarm, so is every other part of the body.

8

THE ACTION OF THE SURVIVAL INSTINCT

Sometimes when I explain about the survival instinct to a patient or a patient's parent, I ask them to imagine that they are in the jungle alone. By putting yourself in this position, you can begin to understand how you behave under stress. Try it for yourself.

Imagine you are lost and hungry and nighttime is approaching. You sense danger all around; larger animals looking for prey and poisonous reptiles lurking in the undergrowth. And less dangerous, but still confronting, biting and stinging insects on the ground, leeches in the water, and mosquitoes in the air. This is not a nice place to be. You are very frightened, so what do you imagine happens next? Do you fall into a calm, relaxed, and invigorating sleep, or do you lie awake hearing every noise and rustle in the trees?

In this state of fight and flight, why do you think you hear every noise no matter how small? Because when your survival instinct is in a state of alarm, it wants to guarantee as best it can that nothing will creep up on you and take you by surprise. When do you imagine that something is most likely to take you by surprise in a dangerous place like the jungle? Answer - at night. So how does your survival instinct protect you from attack? Answer – it sharpens your senses to an almost ridiculous level so you can hear every slither in the underbrush and smell anything that has an odor.

PANDA's kids have heightened senses due to their survival instinct being in fight or flight most of the time. They can hear a whisper from another room or smell anything in your cooking that you are trying to hide. They will refuse or spit out anything distasteful, or refuse to eat anything they don't already know they like. They can be mistrustful of new people and reluctant to make new friends. Many claim that they can smell an odor nearby and you will search the house but you will not find anything. If a PANDAS child has a headache or feels sick, they will often be light sensitive, sometimes even to the point of photophobia. If they are in a flare they may avoid certain textures, or be compelled to touch an object with a texture that gives them comfort.

Case 4
Sarah – female aged 14 years
Sarah's mother had not slept properly in years and she could not remember the last time she slept alone or with her husband in her own bed. With her husband's busy work schedule and looking after Sarah, she had no idea how she and her husband found any time for their relationship.

Sarah could not sleep on her own and she had been this way for as long as her mother could remember. Sarah needed to hold her mother's hand while she slept, but it was too close and uncomfortable for Sarah to have her mother in the bed with her, so every night, Sarah's mother had to sleep on a mattress on the floor next to her daughter, holding her hand as it draped down the side of the bed. She had asked Sarah to meet her half way and at least allow her to buy a double or queen sized bed so she could be more comfortable, but Sarah would have none of it. A double bed was way too big as it made her feel alone and scared. A queen size bed was just out of the question. The more Sarah's mother pleaded her case, the more Sarah resorted to guilt - the last refuge when someone has run out of ideas. 'You don't love me.' 'Why do you want me to suffer?' 'You don't even care about me.' 'I hate you because you hate me!'

Mostly Sarah could not sleep because her mind would not stop racing. She was frightened of someone breaking into the house, but she would also go over the events of her school day wondering whether any of the other girls at school really liked her and whether or not she had said anything that may have upset someone and caused her to have enemies.

Sarah was always worse during her PANDAS flares and it was when her paranoia became almost frantic. However, even outside of her flares, Sarah was highly suspicious by nature and intensely confrontational with everyone in the house. Her parents had all but given up asking Sarah to contribute in any way around the house because of her temper and her brooding rages. Sarah suffered a PANDAS episode on average once a fortnight and usually each flare would last two to three days. Her mother recognized she was in a flare, not only by the intensification of her signs and symptoms, but also how her cheeks would redden and her pupils dilate so massively they would almost cover the whole of her iris.

When Sarah became upset, she was not one of those teenagers who would have an outburst and then it would all be over; Sarah stewed with anger until it turned to hatred. Sarah hated her teachers at school because she knew they didn't like her and she hated her sister and her brother because she believed her parents loved them more than her.

She had no real friends of her own but instead would try and play with her sister's friends whenever they came over to the house. However, that occurrence was becoming less and less as Sarah's sister had stopped inviting her friends, not out of spite, but because it always ended in a fight between Sarah and her sister or between Sarah and her sister's friend. Sarah would take control of whatever game was going on and change the rules or invent new ones that better suited her skills. When the inevitable argument about the game began, it was either Sarah's sister or the friend who would leave because Sarah always refused to move, even if she was in her sister's room.

Everything always had to be done Sarah's way. Her parents had sought the help of all manner of counselors and felt continuously compelled to defend themselves against accusations that they had somehow contributed to, or even caused this behavior by giving in to her demands. Her parents did everything they could do, to not give in to her pressures. Other people assumed that Sarah's personality had been created, spoilt in the traditional sense, by her parents giving her everything she wanted, if she yelled loudly enough. One counsellor concluded that Sarah had learned through trial and error that nastiness eventually would give her what she wanted.

The truth was, both her parents had withdrawn nearly everything Sarah enjoyed in the hope that their discipline would have an effect. They had threatened, then carried out the threat of no longer taking her to her favorite dancing class. They had taken the TV out of her room. They refused to buy her clothes every time she asked, and they had stopped pretending to justify her absences from school; all to no avail. In fact, they admitted that all their punishments had achieved was to make matters worse. Sarah continued to be convinced that everyone hated her.

Sarah also suffered from severe migraines that occurred once a month, just before her cycle. She also suffered with a throbbing type headache at least twice a week and sometimes more often. These headaches were made even worse if she forgot to drink water, which she had to remind herself to do because she claimed to have no thirst impulse. If she ate too many sweets she would get a headache, and if the weather was hot she would also get headaches.

Sarah had a facial tic that looked like a grimace. The best way of describing the look was like sucking on a lemon. She would even have a little head shake or shudder at the end of pulling this face.

At school Sarah was quite well behaved, although she was behind in all her classes. She had been assessed as having normal intelligence. Her parents believed that she was behind with her schooling out of pure stubborn laziness. Her father described her as being the laziest girl imaginable. Sarah's mother was sitting next to her husband while he was saying this to me and I fully expected some sort of defense on Sarah's behalf. It is common in a clinical environment for a mother to try and temper, rather than contradict, any criticism of her child. So I was waiting for her to say something to her husband like, 'Well, yes she can be a little bit slovenly at times but I think the laziest girl in the world is taking things a bit too far.' But Sarah's mother had no interjection, she just nodded in agreement.

In regard to food, if her mother tried to put anything on her plate that even resembled a vegetable or a fruit, Sarah would pick up the vegetable and throw it at her mother's face, screaming how she hates this stuff and not to dare give her anything like that in the future. As a result, her diet was poor; white breads and pasta, a few pieces of chicken, an occasional milk shake, and some fries.

Earlier, I stated that dietary advice is given to patients on a 'do what you can' basis. It is cases like Sarah's that highlight why I do not initially suggest that parents introduce a stricter diet, even when it is clearly required. PANDAS kids burn up energy at a phenomenal rate. Often it seems these kids do so little, so where their ravenous appetite comes from can seem a mystery, but anxiety burns vast amounts of energy, and as a result, the PANDAS palate will always gravitate to high energy foods if that kind of food is available. This means sugary foods and foods rich in refined carbohydrates, such as breads, pastas, cookies, and cakes.

Sarah's mother had stopped buying soft drink because Sarah would consume gallons and then be almost bouncing off the walls, but she hadn't been able to go much further.

Sarah's moods could change at a moment's notice on most days, but if there was strep going around the school, they could change by the hour. She would be laughing one minute while happily playing with her little brother, then suddenly there would be a scream and her brother would run into the room crying with scratch marks down his face. Sarah's school had been asked to notify them whenever strep was going around.

Sarah would often feel sick to her stomach, especially during a PANDAS flare, and many times her mother would comfort her while she vomited so much that after a while, only bile was coming up. Every gastric test had been done but no test ever revealed a specific problem.

Her sleep was restless even with her mother present. She would groan in her dreams and jerk and thrash about. About once a week, Sarah would leap out of bed with cramping in her leg. The cramps were always in her left leg, in her calf muscle.

I was lucky with Sarah because I got her remedy right first time. That isn't always the case.

After a month on her remedy, her parents stated that her behavior had improved dramatically. Within the first month of treatment the number of outbursts had decreased noticeably. Her temper tantrums, which had been almost daily before the remedy had decreased to every few days. The intensity of her anger had also decreased but not as much, from 10/10 to 7/10. Her anger was still apparent, but when she did get angry, it was not to the same degree. No-one suffered any scratch marks that month.

Sarah experienced a PANDAS flare within a short time of commencing treatment but there was a noticeable difference. According to her mother, she had shown all the signs of getting the flare, that is, feeling sick, flushed in the cheeks, with wildly dilated pupils, but Sarah's behavior did not worsen dramatically. After a day or two she seemed to return to normal, which was an improvement. Because she only experienced one flare for the month and not the expected two, we can add to her improvement a fifty percent reduction in PANDAS flares.

This alone would have been a good enough reason to keep going with the same remedy, but there were other improvements as well. Sarah had not complained anywhere near as much about her stomach during the last flare, nor had she vomited, even though she experienced some nausea.

Her period had come and gone, and while she still ended up in bed with a migraine, it was not as bad as she was used to. The migraine which had been 10/10 before the remedy was 7/10 this time.

More importantly was the fact that Sarah had not been having any consistent headaches during the week.

In regards to her sleep, there has been no real change, although Sarah's mother did think that perhaps she was sleeping a little more peacefully. There had also been no change to her diet because her mother did not feel she was ready to try and introduce anything new at that early stage.

I continued to treat Sarah with the same remedy for another month and at the end of the next month Sarah was still feeling better. Her parents both agreed there had been continued improvement and that the house was far more relaxed than it used to be. Sarah's moods were far more stable and she was not flying off the handle at the drop of a hat.

Sarah had not missed a day of school in the last month, which was highly unusual. She did have one headache but it had now been two months since her twice a week regular headaches. During her period, she also had a headache but she did not have a migraine. This was the first time that she did not have a migraine at all, before or during her period, since her periods began.

Sarah and her sister still had a couple of fights, but nowhere near to the same degree, and once Sarah even admitted that she was wrong and apologized after cooling down. She was having less outbursts overall and the intensity was down to 4 or 5 out of 10.

There had still been no change to Sarah's diet and she had not made any close friends. But on the positive side, Sarah's need to control and dictate every activity and every discussion with her brother and sister had eased. So too had Sarah's need to be the center of attention every time her sister had a friend over to play.

Two months after this follow up, four months after starting her remedy, Sarah has joined a basketball team. By the end of each game, she was red faced and panting because she wasn't fit yet, but everyone has to start somewhere. I see this desire to both move and mix with other people as a great step forward, so I was very happy with this progress. As well as her decision to become more fit, she also voluntarily asked her mother about weight management and diet.

Sarah was not grossly overweight, but she was heavier than she should be. Sarah's mother had discussed with Sarah a number of ideas, which we had already spoken about in regards to diet, being careful not to mention that she had taken this information from me.

A number of PANDAS kids are highly suspicious and get extremely angry if they think other people are talking about them. Even though Sarah was improving, her mother was still cautious.

PANDAS kids are often embarrassed about having PANDAS. Many hate it with a passion. They don't want to talk about it and they don't want anyone else to know. Some don't mind sharing their symptoms with a discrete practitioner and their mother or father but that's usually their limit. Some won't even share that much. They tell a little to their mother but what they share is limited. A very few I have have treated enjoy their PANDAS because they feel it separates them from others, like a kind of specialness or individuality that a normal kid doesn't have. However, this feeling of special fondness is rare.

During her next consultation her mother shared that Sarah still had not had a migraine with any of her periods and almost no headaches – unlike the weekly frequency prior to the remedy. Sarah has not had what her mother would regard as a full blown PANDAS flare since she started treatment. Even though she has had the occasional sore throat and even a cold, her signs and symptoms stayed pretty typical of a normal cold and did not advance into the PANDAS flare she was bracing herself for. Sarah's pupils had even returned to their normal size and had not dilated since treatment began.

Sarah's mother still said that the house had to adapt to some of Sarah's moods but she believed that was just her personality and the type of person she is. However, in regards to temper outbursts with brooding and violence, there had been none in the last few months. Sarah was getting along well – for the most part – with her sister and would even spend a little bit of time with her brother.

When I questioned her about her daughter's separation anxiety, she said Sarah no longer needed to hang on to her when they went out, in fact she didn't even give her the time of day, so typical of too cool for school girls her age.

By the next consultation, Sarah had made a couple of friends on her basketball team and even had one of them over to her place for a practice session. This same friend also asked Sarah over for a sleep-over to which she nervously agreed. In preparation for the big night, Sarah asked if her mother would not sleep with her a couple of times to see if she would be okay alone. Sarah's mother calmly agreed to give it go and suppressed her desire to jump up and click her heels.

Two nights that first week, Sarah slept through the night on her own without waking, which gave her the confidence to state that she did not think she needed her mother to sleep next to her anymore.

At the dinner table, not every meal was plain pasta and bread and Sarah had begun to eat some lettuce, apple, banana, and even a bit of hidden broccoli with her pasta. It was a start. One important point to share is that when her mother did try to hide vegetables other than broccoli into the pasta, Sarah still didn't eat it, but she didn't throw it at her mother or scream at her. She simply moved it to one side of her plate and when her mother asked if she was going to eat it 'because it's good for you', Sarah would reply 'maybe later'. Now every parent knows 'I'll eat it later,' really means no but at least she was tactful.

Sarah is still under my care with less frequent follow ups, a few times a year. As a footnote, Sarah still sleeps alone every night without her mother needing to be in the same room.

For Homeopaths
The rubrics I chose for Sarah's repertorisation were -

> MIND; FEAR; alone, of being (80)
> MIND; THOUGHTS; persistent (100)
> EYE; PUPILS; dilated (188)
> MIND; HATRED (52)
> GENERALITIES; MENSES; agg.; before (109)
> HEAD PAIN; PULSATING, throbbing (217)
> STOMACH; VOMITING; General (439)
> SLEEP; RESTLESS (408)

Sarah's facial analysis placed her in the yellow color group (Psora) which means she has the type of defense system that protects the core by throwing any invading virus or bacteria out on to the surface. In Sarah's case this also included her emotional stress. The remedy I chose was Pulsatilla 30C given once daily.

Pulsatilla is a yellow remedy which means it's action has the same outward force as Sarah's immune system. This means I am doubling up on how Sarah's body likes to heal and balance itself. Pulsatilla 30 C once daily, was constantly repeated because of her progressive and lasting improvement.

9

SENSITIVITY AND OVER-REACTION

So many PANDAS kids are either sensitive to, or allergic to, a variety of foods, and it seems the longer the PANDAS has been in their lives, the more allergies they have. Sensitivity means you can have some of the same responses as a food allergy, but because a sensitivity does generate a systemic immune response like an allergy does, the signs and symptoms are generally less severe, and certainly don't last as long. Some say the only way to really tell the difference is to have a blood test to see if specific foods cause a measurable immune reaction, and that might be so, but an easier way, although it is hardly fool proof, is to monitor your child's response to a suspect food every time they have it. If they drink milk, and sometimes (but not necessarily every time) have a negative response, or they can tolerate dairy in a different form, for example they can't drink milk but they can eat ice cream, then they would have a dairy sensitivity rather than an allergy.

Why does all this make a difference anyway? Because often you will find that your child's food sensitivities will start fading away, or at least diminishing, as successful treatment continues. At the beginning of treatment your PANDAS child may be sensitive to sugar and gluten, but by the end of successful treatment many PANDAS kids can have some sugar or a little gluten and not go off the rails. It doesn't mean they can make these sensitive foods a staple part of their diet, but they will have less reaction and so won't feel as socially isolated.

I mentioned earlier that dietary advice was an important factor in the treatment of PANDAS, but it may not be the type of dietary advice you might expect. Often naturopaths like to put clients on rigid, specifically controlled diets such as the GAPS diet for PANDAS kids, and I can tell you right now that a lot of parents have claimed reasonable improvements from this diet. However, I have never seen diet alone make the kind of changes I have seen treating PANDAS with HFA homeopathy, improved diet and better exercise.

I spoke about being lost in the jungle and how the nervous response would be heightened, to explain why some PANDAS kids have the signs and symptoms they do. However, there is more to understand about a system that is in constant fight or flight. It is not just the nervous system that becomes hyper responsive.

It is the job of the brain to keep the mind and the body coordinated and harmonious; the body cannot be in a different place to the mind. However, the mind and body pathway is not just a one-way street. The mind will also start to feel the same way as the body. If the nervous system is in a state of fight or flight, it is only a matter of time before that same sense of agitation, nervousness, and inability to rest, become a constant part of your PANDAS child's demeanor. More than that, the nervous system cannot be in a state of turmoil while the rest of the body is in a state of peace and tranquility. If your child's nervous system is tense, reactive, and hyper-responsive, then so too will many other parts of their body, especially the immune and the digestive system.

I know a lot of practitioners will see this the other way around, that is, the already existing gut problems are causing the nervous system to respond in a negative over-stimulated way, but after treating many PANDAS kids I think there is more going on.

Of course it would make my treatment plan easy (as a naturopath) if the gut came before the nervous system, which in turn came before the mental state, but with PANDAS, I believe the digestive system is going out in sympathy because of a nervous/immune dysfunction.

PANDAS is a syndrome, which means in the simplest of terms, that the entire system is out of balance. It also means that a total and holistic approach must be employed. By holistic, I don't mean the more typical fragmented holism where one remedy is given for digestion along with a herb for the nervous system and another to try and bring some comfort to a troubled mind. A true holistic approach has to be something that recognizes the constitution as a complete totality, and this is where homeopathy comes into its own. I will discuss homeopathy in greater depth shortly, but for now I want to continue with diet and lifestyle.

PANDAS kids generally have a nervous system that reacts to everything. Is it really stretching our thinking too far, to believe that this over-reaction flows on to other areas of the body? Over-reaction is a conditioned constitutional state. It explains why PANDAS kids also have immune systems that react to every germ and weather condition, and why PANDAS kids have digestive systems that over-react to a wide range of foods and additives.

If we can stop or slow down this generalized over-reactive trend, this condition for the most part, will be calmed considerably, including the over-reactive, hyper-responsive mind. There is a caveat to this statement; the calming down of this PANDAS over-reaction applies primarily to those children, to whom PANDAS is the major or the only problem. Some kids and teens have PANDAS alone, while others have PANDAS as a co-factor to more severe and consistent psychiatric problems. I will refer to the PANDAS alone child as belonging to group one and the child with PANDAS alongside a psychiatric disorder as group two.

The distinction between these two groups is vast, both in day to day life and in their potential to be stabilized. A typical PANDAS child (group one) is one where, for most of the time, there is nothing really wrong with their behavior either socially or intellectually until a PANDAS flare takes place. This flare can give an unsuspecting parent a huge fright as they watch their normally rational child become increasingly out of control, in either their temper, their OCD, their fears, or all of the above.

Children who have PANDAS as an overlay on top of other psychiatric conditions (group two) have a demeanor that is generally out of step with others, or their behavior is deemed to be more socially unacceptable or at the very least more socially unaware; some can even be delusional.

The difference between group one kids and group two, is that group two kids suffer these symptoms almost constantly. Sure these group two kids might have pockets of clarity or times when they don't seem quite as bad, but when reviewed over a long period of time, their delusions or their fantasies are a constant trend and always exist to a greater or lesser degree. PANDAS, for these group two kids, simply means that their condition becomes noticeably worse if they become physically sick, stressed or tired, or eat too many incorrect foods. After the illness or stress is over, they return back to their normal or usual behavior pattern. However, normalcy for these group two children after their flare is not the same normalcy as that of group one. Normal for group one, means no appreciable difference in age appropriate behavior to the majority of other kids around them. Normal for group two generally means a return to what is normal for them.

The subdivision into two different groups is important to understand in reference to my treatment prognosis. The more consistently a group of signs and symptoms present in a child, the more entrenched and difficult they are to influence. Meaning, the more a child displays a certain set of behaviors, the longer and slower the treatment plan will be. If a child comes from group one, that is, they are generally fine except during a flare, then I would expect to see a reasonably quick response in that child. Allowing for individual variables, I would expect a child from group one to respond positively to my treatment within five consultations or less. If the child comes from the group two category, it is impossible to put a time frame on treatment response, and it is just as difficult to know before treatment to what extent they will respond. The majority will respond in some positive way, but just how much and when – that is unpredictable.

10

PANDAS AND FOOD

Getting any child to eat properly in today's day and age is difficult, but getting a child with behavioral problems, especially during a PANDAS flare, to eat natural whole foods is pretty much bordering on impossible. Particularly when you remember that a large part of the PANDAS syndrome includes symptoms of oppositional defiance. This is why, when it comes to diet, all my suggestions are given in the spirit of, 'do the best you can.' Of course this becomes easier once treatment brings about balance, but even balanced kids will push parents to supply them with junk. The 21st century parent may have more mod cons than ever before, but the authority to feed their children properly has been undermined by fast food peddlers.

If your PANDAS child simply refuses to eat well, or in some cases, eat anything you provide, don't worry too much at the beginning; diet is important but it is not a prerequisite for improvement. It is not a situation where if the diet is wrong all else will fail, but it certainly makes the road to recovery steeper and more strenuous.

In saying that, there is yet another caveat, and that is the constant eating of refined sugar in any of its forms. PANDAS kids already have an over-reactive system. The last thing they need is a lot of refined sugar adding to their problems.

Some doctors will disagree with the idea that sugar contributes to negative behavior, citing studies like one written in the

New England Journal of Medicine titled: 'Effects of Diets High in Sucrose or Aspartame on The Behavior and Cognitive Performance of Children,' which claimed that children do not go crazy after a sugar binge, and that they do not react badly to colorings and flavorings. All I can say is that study obviously did not involve any PANDAS children because those finding simply do not apply. Another so-called 'dispelled myth' that does not apply to PANDAS kids is their relationship to phases of the moon. Scientific studies written in journals such as Scientific American in February 2009 claim that any relationship between moon phases and behavior is absolute nonsense. That study group is another group that must have been PANDAS free.

Regardless of what studies like these state, the fact is, I meet parents from all over the world and they tell me similar stories. In fact, far too similar to be ignored, which is why I want to share them. If you believe that your PANDAS child is definitely more uncontrollable in their behavior after sugar, then you are not alone. If you feel as if your PANDAS child is definitely worse during one of the moon phases, because the timing of their flares always seems to coincide with a moon cycle, don't feel strange, many PANDAS parents have noticed the exact same thing.

There are lots of different diets that claim good results for different conditions. I have already mentioned the GAPS diet that is said to be beneficial to patients with seizures and other neurological problems, and many of my patients would agree with this claim. So if you already have your PANDAS child on a specific diet tailored for their condition, and that diet seems to be helping, then don't change a thing. However, diet can be a little hit and miss when it comes to getting continuous results.

Some physicians say the best way to understand the body is to see it as a machine. But that philosophy leaves out many factors. Your car, for example, is a machine, but it is not an interactive sentient being; it does not judge, sense, react, or favor. But human beings do. Our mind, brain, senses, and body, are all highly responsive to what is going on around us. We are not machines; we are people. The treatment of a human being involves many more factors than mechanics.

The whole purpose of any medical system is to get people well. Medicine, in any form, serves no other function. However, some practitioners seem to get lost and start thinking that it's more important to stay faithful to their science or their medical ideology than it is to get their patients' well. Being true to veganism or to the Paleolithic diet becomes a bigger issue than the people they were setting out to help in the first place.

As a PANDAS parent, you have only one task and that is to get your child as well and as balanced as possible. If that is by homeopathy, that's great. If it is by conventional medicine, Chinese medicine, or faith healing – whatever works is ok, as long your child is getting better. Diet has a special place as an aid to treatment and it can be significant for some, so I want to explore it further.

After years of learning about food and diets, trialling diets myself, and hearing from patients about every type of diet imaginable – from the successful to the absurd - I keep my diet philosophy simple. In fact, my whole dietary attitude is simple for everybody, not just PANDAS kids, and that philosophy is to keep your food as natural and as whole as possible, and to keep any food that had been refined to the barest minimum – and that is it. Four years of naturopathic college and nearly a quarter of a century of experience and in the end it is as simple as that.

If you have a food allergy, then keep away from that food. If you have multiple food sensitivities, then you need to understand that it is not the foods that are causing you (or your PANDAS child) the biggest problem; it is the imbalance in your system (or their system). Once you get the body back into balance and start to regenerate health, you will find that the impact of a number of food sensitivities will also begin to become less and less dominant. This doesn't always mean they will go away altogether, although for many people they do. Often, it becomes about quantity, that is keeping the intake of that particular food to a minimum; don't expect a previously sensitive food to become a staple of your child's diet.

The diet of everyone, regardless of their ailments and complaints, should always consist of at least ninety percent whole natural foods and no more than ten percent splurge. Anything in a packet is a splurge. Anything that comes with a nutritional label should also be regarded as a splurge. Anything bought in a bakery is a splurge, and so too is anything that comes out of a can.

As a PANDAS parent, if you don't know already, wheat products can be very upsetting to a number of PANDAS kids and also too much fruit – even though they are both whole foods. Dairy can also be an issue because there is often a lot of congestion and stuffiness in a PANDAS child due to their sensitivities and allergies. So adding anymore congestion in the form of foods like milk or cream, can sometimes be too much for their system to tolerate. Too much dairy may result in headaches, sinus problems, or continuous colds.

So when beginning treatment and while sensitivities still exist, it is best to keep your PANDAS child on the restricted diet you think is best, or if they are not on any restricted diet as yet, be prepared to make some small but positive changes. Start by reducing all refined sugars as best you can. Refined sugar is any type of sugar that comes in a packet, soft drink can, a bar of chocolate, or a packaged cake or sweet.

As treatment continues and progress moves forward, especially once your PANDAS child's mood, behavior, and OCD symptoms begin to calm and come under control, you may be able to give them some dietary leeway, especially if your child has been invited to a party. I have already discussed how your child is not just a machine, and social acceptance is equally as important as the type of food they eat – but only once their moods are under control.

The biggest culprit for out of control behavior is often the soft drinks or sodas – depending on which country you live in. These fizzy drinks can push PANDAS kids to the edge, so you want to make sure, if you are going to allow them the freedom to have these drinks every now and then so they don't feel left out, to make sure their signs and symptoms have been under control and that their behavior has been stable for a while. Even if you do allow them to splurge, remember, we are only talking about sugar as a very irregular treat. It cannot play a daily part in their diet or problems will continue or start again.

Why is it so important to keep food as natural and whole as possible, and what is whole anyway? First of all, natural does not mean that the word natural is printed somewhere on the food label. Such as *natural colors* or *all natural preservatives* or - you have to love this spin – *made originally from natural products*. Natural means food that is grown in the ground or picked from a tree, or as fresh as possible from an animal. There is zero to little factory processing in a natural food.

Apart from the occasional plastic wrapper, there is no processing in a pumpkin. By contrast, there can be quite a lot of various food processes in a can of pumpkin soup. Eating an apple or an orange creates a vastly different reaction in the body to eating an apple or orange flavored sweet. Eating a freshly cooked shrimp or prawn, depending on which country you live in, shares very little in common with eating a shrimp or prawn flavored cracker. A PANDAS digestive system, or any digestive system for that matter, has adapted and is used to the proteins contained within fresh shrimp. As a food source this type of fresh protein can be easily digested. These proteins are not what you get when you munch into a prawn cracker. In fact, most of the time the closest thing to a real shrimp or prawn is the picture on the packet. A natural diet is also vital for keeping your PANDAS child's system as chemical free as possible.

The digestive system of your PANDAS child is the product of hundreds of thousands of years of adaptation that now enables the gut to process easily whatever is natural. Remember, the link between all PANDAS symptoms is over-reaction, so there is a much greater likelihood that a PANDAS child will over-react to a food that contains new or foreign unrecognized chemicals, than to a food that has been around for a hundred thousand years.

The term 'whole food' means the same as natural, in the sense that we are talking about an original and complete food. This means eating an apple rather than drink a concentrated apple juice or eating a banana, orange or some berries rather than taking a vitamin C tablet. The whole food and the processed version are not the same thing. If you want to take extra vitamin C as well as the fruit then that is a different issue, but don't ever think that taking a pill is as good as eating a whole food.

Case 5
Thomas – male aged 16 years.
When Thomas first came to me as a patient he was allergic to almost everything. What started out as a few seasonal hay fever symptoms only a few years earlier had developed progressively into an array of sensitivities and allergies to almost every pollen known to humankind. His allergies involved such a wide range of foods that finding something to eat became a full time job for Thomas' mother.

Thomas could not eat anything artificial as the colorings or the added flavorings would make his eyes swell up and redden. If there were pesticides on his vegetables or fruit, he would have nausea and/or negative behavioral changes. If Thomas ate wheat, he would become aggressive. If he had eggs he would get a throbbing headache, and dairy would make him feel as if he were about to get a flu. Eating salt hurt his tongue, and sugar excited all his fears and brought out his worst behavior, so that he rarely ate anything sweet at all.

If Thomas went to the park, he would end up with hives. If he swam in a chlorinated pool, he would get an ear infection, and salt from the sea made Thomas' skin crack open. If an insect bit him, he would spend the next day sick and swollen in bed.

On top of Thomas' allergy symptoms were his OCD and PANDAS behavior. When Thomas' fears were at their worst, his aggressive behaviors were also heightened, although his mother never knew the exact triggers for these episodes. For a while she thought the cause was a strep infection, but then she decided this could not be because his tests showed up negative for strep. She began to wonder whether Thomas' behavior was linked to moon phases but again ruled this connection out, as no pattern could be observed.

When Thomas was in a flare, his fears were dominated by terrifying thoughts regarding the supernatural. He also had fears regarding people breaking into the house, but the supernatural fears were the worst. During a flare he would hear voices calling to him; they would not compel him to do things, nor would they tell him how bad he was, they just called his name or said single words. Thomas was tested for schizophrenia – and was found not to be schizophrenic. Sometimes Thomas would see a vision of someone watching him. The people in these visions were indistinct so he did not recognize any of them but they would always give him a fright. Thankfully, his visions were never malevolent.

Many parents ask whether I think these visions and auditory hallucinations are real or just part of disturbed mind due to a PANDAS flare. The bottom line is I do not really know. I am practical enough that I do not accept that every vision has some supernatural connection, but I am also open enough to understand that there is more going on with some children that I can possibly fathom. However, if a PANDAS child only sees or hears supernatural voices when they are in a flare, I would question the legitimacy of those voices. I am not questioning whether they actually see or hear the person or voice - of that I am certain - but I question whether a real supernatural connection has been made.

On the other hand, there are many PANDAS kids that claim to witness spirits or hear voices outside of times when they are in a flare. Thomas was unusual as he fell into the category of a bit of both. He would see people indistinctly in his vision when he was well, but he would be more scared and hear loud voices when he was in a flare.

On average, Thomas would flare for three or four days every two weeks.

Apart from his allergies and his consistent flares, Thomas was a normal well-balanced kid. He had a healthy vibrant social life and was well liked by his friends. He played sports and had recently started a relationship with his first girlfriend. Thomas did reasonably well at school with not much effort; his passions were more social than academic.

Thomas was first put on Arsenicum 30 C daily, but there was little improvement. After a reassessment of his miasm (through facial analysis) a second remedy was chosen, Belladonna 30 C daily, and Thomas began to improve.

Under the second remedy, the distance between PANDAS flares began to improve. Instead of every two weeks, Thomas experienced flares every three to four weeks and then with much less intensity. After a few months of treatment – almost exclusively homeopathic, as his mother was well read and experienced with diet and nutrition - his flares had extended to once every three months, and even then only when he was sick with some sort of virus.

What makes Thomas' case equally important as the reduction in flares, is the change in his sensitivities, especially to food. He continued to improve dramatically as each month passed. Not only his physical symptoms and behavior improved, with each step forward, his body repaired and strengthened itself. It was clear he was building strength because the time between flares kept extending, and the triggers that usually brought on an episode needed to be stronger to elicit any type of negative response. When the body is weakened and in a continuous or at least semi-continuous state of imbalance, a PANDAS flare can occur over the smallest of triggers.

The more out of balance a PANDAS child is, the more strongly and consistently they react and flare. In addition, the more they flare, the more their energy gets disturbed and the more drained or hyperactive they become. The more drained of energy or the more scattered and hyperactive they become, the less chance their body has of repairing any damage caused by those flares, fevers, and allergies. The more damage that is done, the greater the sensitivity to their triggers, and around and around it goes. The only way to get on top of this merry-go-round is to rebuild the body so it is less reactive and the opposite cycle can occur. The less reactive and sensitive your PANDAS child becomes the more energy their body has to heal and repair itself.

PANDA'S kids are like a house in a storm. The weaker the house, the less of a storm it takes to cause damage. However, once their house is strong, all the little things that used to push them over the edge begin to fall to the wayside. This does not mean that after treatment, PANDAS children are invulnerable to every germ or allergen going around, but it does mean they should be able to eat a sweet or indulge in some junk food at a party, and not suffer the consequences for days.

By the time Thomas was well and truly out of the woods from his continuous flares, he not only could eat sugar on the odd occasion without suffering, but he could also eat fruit again as a staple part of his diet, without consequences. In addition, his happy mother reported no more fears of the supernatural, no more visions, no hives, and only a few minor ear infections, which quickly resolved.

After a year of treatment, the only continuing weakness for Thomas was if he pushed himself too much, for example with a series of late nights. That was still his Achilles heel. All kids get a little grumpy and unapproachable when they are tired, but Thomas would get beyond just a little grumpy by the third or fourth late night. His behavior would begin to be like his previous PANDAS flares – usually not as bad as when he first came to me, but getting close.

What this shows is that even though homeopathic remedies are highly effective, a total approach that encompasses diet, exercise, sleep, and relaxation, is still required for the best results.

Will Thomas ever be able to live it up and eat pizza and other junk food on a regular basis? Let me answer by saying that no one should be living on junk food day after day, week after week. PANDAS is irrelevant to this advice. Every person, regardless of who they are or what weaknesses they have, will be under stress if junk food is the foundation of their diet.

To understand PANDAS properly you have to see yourself or your child as having an inbuilt set of scales, with energy levels on one side and their signs and symptoms on the other side. When the body starts to get exhausted and run down, like it does with too much junk food or too many late nights, weak areas of the body begin to show characteristic signs and symptoms.

This model is true for everyone, irrespective of his or her condition or weakness. If you were born with a propensity to liver problems, those problems will magnify when you are stressed, depleted, or tired for too long. This is the key; stress is far more than just being emotionally upset. Stress needs to be understood as a state or outcome that takes our energy levels out of homeostasis. Junk food wears down the body's energy because junk food takes more energy to digest than the energy it gives back. Chronic junk food consumption equals a chronic depletion of energy, which in turn equals a chronic state of stress. PANDA's kids do not do well under any stress because they already have an over-reactive system.

Sleep deprivation is also as draining and stressful to the body as eating too much junk food, however with sleep loss the effects will show themselves even sooner.

For Homeopaths
The rubrics I chose for Thomas' case were -

>GENERALITIES; SENSITIVENESS (187)
>MIND; DELUSIONS, imaginations; voices, hears (53)
>MIND; FEAR; ghosts, of (41)
>SKIN; ERUPTIONS; urticaria (210)

Once again, Thomas' case shows the importance of accurate photo taking and analysis. In my first facial analysis, I had misinterpreted some of his facial features, which is why he did not respond to the Arsenicum, even though it was a well repertorised remedy. Thomas' facial structure showed that his defense response belonged to the purple group (syco-syphilitic). Arsenicum is not a (HFA) purple remedy. Arsenicum may still help to a degree because it is a well repertorised remedy, but history tells me that it's positive effects will not hold for very long nor will it repeat well, even if I increased the potency.

Whenever a patient does not respond to a remedy, the first thing I do is recheck my facial analysis. I am so confident in this system that I know that if I have the facial analysis right, it is only a matter of time before I get the remedy right. Selection based on symptom totality without the miasmatic indicator means it can take a lot longer to find an accurate remedy. Sometimes the facial analysis is correct but the remedy just doesn't resonate, so I recheck the totality of the case, re-repertorise, and find a new remedy within the same group. In Thomas' case, re-checking his facial structure showed that my mistake was that I selected the wrong miasm. The new selection of Belladonna (also a well repertorised remedy), but this time a remedy that had the same defensive action as Thomas, made all the difference and he began to respond immediately.

Thomas' case also shows the importance of being patient and of the practitioner being able to evaluate symptoms in order to know when to change and when to keep going with a remedy. Belladonna 30C was given to Thomas once a day.

11

DIETS AND BACTERIA

When a PANDAS child is out of balance, even a spoonful of sugar can have disastrous consequences. Once they are back in balance, they are fine to go to a party every now and then without a week of hell as the aftermath, but no one – healthy or otherwise – can eat too much sugar or lose too much sleep for too long. This is all common sense, however, as the French writer Voltaire once pointed out, 'Common sense is not so common.'

The essentials for optimal health are the same things that will keep your symptoms at bay. Symptoms go down when health goes up; it is that simple.

So if that is the case, why we do we need medicine of any kind? Because the above statement, 'health up equals symptoms down' only applies to a body that is balanced and strong in the first place. When the body is out of balance, everything goes haywire. The energy from food is not utilized properly, the immune system can start attacking everything it sees (including itself) without discrimination, emotions and thoughts become scattered, changing disproportionately to the circumstances around them.

When we are in this state, we are not able to heal ourselves, even with the right food and conditions, because the body's energy is going to all the wrong places. Nature's healing program is wonderful but it has its own limitations. A fever can easily turn into a febrile convulsion, and when it does, the resulting convulsion becomes more dangerous than the infection it was originally trying to prevent. Nature's healing capabilities are much better suited to healthy balanced bodies than unhealthy or out of balanced systems. Perhaps this is a by-product that comes from nature's striving demand for survival of the fittest, a legacy of a natural system that is trying to cull any weaknesses from the species. Whatever the reason, the reality is clear; it is easier to stay well than it is to get well.

Getting well requires far more energy and effort than lifestyle changes alone can provide and this is especially seen with PANDAS. Some sort of medicine, homeopathic or otherwise, is a vital requirement for any system under stress.

Healthy eating is easy, if that is what you know and follow, but advice in the form of a diet is common and often the starting point back to natural healthy eating. There are a few different diets' that parent's claim help their PANDAS child, so a quick review of healthy eating is worthwhile.

Gluten Free Diet
Wheat and other gluten containing grains, have been a naturopathic suspect in a number of psychological and emotional disorders for decades. In fact, long before gluten free was even close to becoming common, naturopaths were cautioning patient's about being aware of too many grains in their diet. This was in case they had a sensitivity; alternative medicine and alternative thinking is often ahead of the crowd.

However, one has to be open-minded, because naturopathic advice can often be contrary to 'generally accepted' information, particularly when the naturopathic advice is not in the best interest of business or government channels. Alternative ways of solving problems are often not economically what industry wants to hear. Parents seeking the best advice for their children have to weigh up all the information independently - especially in regard to who is paying for studies and whether the outcome has been compromised.

When a naturopath talks about gluten sensitivity or perhaps a gluten intolerance, they are not necessarily claiming that you or your PANDAS child has the organic diagnosis of celiac disease. Gluten sensitivity is distinct and separate from celiac disease and it is far more common. With celiac disease, the villi of the small intestine (villi absorb the nutrients from food) can actually atrophy (shrivel and die), plus there is the presence of a specific antibody that alerts the physician to the fact that something is wrong. Gluten sensitive patients may have none of these celiac hallmarks and yet still react to gluten, or just wheat products generally, in a highly negative way.

Gluten is a mixture of two proteins found in a number of cereal grains, and in people who are sensitive, it can cause what is commonly called a leaky gut. The villi of the small intestine do not completely atrophy, but they do decrease and they decrease in their function, which causes some intestinal space.

There should be no spaces in the small intestine. Inside the body there is yet another protein called Zonulin. It is found in the digestive tract and its job is to keep the cells of the gut tight. However, it is suspected that in some people – PANDAS kids included – that when gluten is combined with Zonulin, it tells this protein to open, rather than to keep the intestinal wall tight. This means that for certain people, gluten will be able to pass through the wall of the small intestine and escape into the blood stream, rather than being contained in the small intestine, where it is safe, and where it belongs.

The immune system operates to a simple premise. Our world and everything in it is divided into two camps of recognition; self and non-self. Self is accepted, good, and left alone to do its thing. Non-self is not accepted, and recognized as bad, and then attacked vigorously in a do or die struggle. The immune system knows no other way. As with all aspects of the physical body, the immune system is run by a program that cannot be reasoned with.

Gluten, in the gut of a healthy person who can tolerate it, is broken down into its most basic components. The nutrients released are distributed as vitamins, minerals, and proteins, to various areas of the body. Gluten is fine, provided it stays in the gut and is broken down in the gut. But if gluten escapes into the blood stream because of its interaction with Zonulin, the immune system is activated because it knows that gluten is foreign to the blood stream. The gluten is regarded as non-self and it must be eliminated. This is what a naturopath means when they say that your PANDAS child has a gluten sensitivity, which is triggering a systemic immune response.

It could be argued that eliminating gluten floating in the blood stream is not a bad thing in itself. That is true, except a continuous immune response caused by constantly eating products containing gluten creates inflammation and cellular damage. The blood brain barrier is a highly selective permeable barrier that separates the circulating blood supply from the brain and the central nervous system. It is the Berlin Wall (for those old enough to remember the Berlin Wall) of the body, designed to let in only specific molecules desired by the brain, such as glucose, oxygen, and certain amino acids, and to keep out anything that might be potentially harmful to this most delicate of body organs. The blood brain barrier achieves its aim by making sure any gaps in its wall are kept tightly closed and sealed.

As already mentioned, one of the proteins the body uses to keep the blood brain barrier tight and without leaks is Zonulin. There is speculation, that if the combination of Zonulin and gluten can cause openings and leaks in the gut, perhaps this same combination (remember gluten due to a leaky gut is now circulating around the body and coming into contact with the blood brain barrier) is causing leaks and holes in the blood brain barrier. This would turn gluten from a protein found in certain grains, into a dangerous inflammatory neurotoxin. Many experts say, and it is a difficult argument to dispute, that PANDAS is caused by an inflammation of the brain and central nervous system, or at least specific parts of it. Therefore, any inflammatory agent, especially one that can cross the blood brain barrier, needs to be avoided.

Assuming the cerebellum and/or the basal ganglia are the areas of the brain subject most to this inflammation, then we would expect other functions controlled by the either cerebellum or the basal ganglia to become disrupted and, depending on the degree of inflammation, to become erratic. The cerebellum is the part of the brain that controls motor movements. The cerebellum helps regulates speech and other voluntary movements such as balance and coordination.

This is interesting on its own to parents of PANDAS kids who suffer from delayed speech, tics, or convulsive movements. What is even more interesting, is how the latest information regarding the cerebellum also shows that it contributes to cognitive processing and emotional regulation.

Is there any specific evidence to know beyond a shadow of doubt that gluten is *a* major or even *the* major culprit behind PANDAS and all its symptoms? The short answer is No. However, there is enough evidence to assume that there is a definite aggravating inflammation going on somewhere in the brain or central nervous system. We also know this by how many PANDAS kids have their behavior temporarily calmed by the use of antibiotics or anti-inflammatory medication.

The scientific studies are not yet finalized, but gluten is on the list of suspects until further investigation reveals otherwise. The most common sources of gluten include, wheat, rye, barley, brewer's yeast, and malt. Rice does not contain gluten, nor do potatoes. Rice is an important substitute for those who like to eat grain based meals. Potatoes are also gluten free and while corn contains a type of gluten, it is usually a type that is better tolerated.

Paleolithic Diet

Also known as the Paleo diet, this way of eating is one of, if not the biggest, dietary rage of modern times, and theoretically it makes sense. At the heart of the argument is the idea that our digestive system evolves to accommodate the foods we eat most often. However, gut evolution, like all evolution, is an extremely slow process. This means the foods that we have traditionally eaten for the longest period of time, will also be the foods that are the most tolerated. They will be the foods that are more nutritionally beneficial, because our system has learned how to utilize every part of these foods. It makes sense that relative new comers to the human diet are not as well tolerated, and not as well utilized, because our digestive system has not had enough time to learn all the tricks of the digestive trade. This is why Paleo supporters stress the importance of eating meat, fats, fruits, and vegetables liberally, and limiting dairy, and assorted grains, including wheat.

Who knows exactly how long human beings have been walking on the face of the earth, when you add our evolutionary predecessors to homo sapiens and their long genetic/digestive lineage. According to the experts, we were making rudimentary tools two or three million years ago. These tools were designed for cutting and crushing, which leads to the belief that we were hunting large animals for meat. The oldest shell middens may go back 140,000 years, but that does not really tell us how long human beings have been eating seafood, just how long ago that one group of people sat around eating shell fish as a tribe. We can assume eating fish and other assorted seafood has been going on for longer than 140,000 years.

Our oldest eating pattern and therefore the one to which we are most biologically adapted, and the oldest by quite a long way, is the consumption of fruit and vegetables. We may have always been omnivorous as a species, but eating bugs and the occasional small catch is hardly meat-eating as we understand it today. Humans need tools to hunt, so eating meat as we currently understand it, could only occur after the appropriate tools were developed and that was two to three million years ago. By contrast, the first known humans to be walking around on two legs were doing so around six million years ago.

So it would seem that fruits, vegetables, and selected seeds, along with a very small proportion of insects and meat, have been consumed for as long as six million years. Bigger portions of meat taken from larger animals have been a part of our diet for around two to three million years. Wheat consumption and wheat as an agricultural crop dates back only ten to twelve thousand years, and rice is roughly the same. Dairy consumption developed a little later; around nine thousand years ago.

Paleolithic advocates are not saying that wheat and dairy are bad in themselves. They highlight the fact that while both these foods may contain a number of essential nutrients, our ability to process these foods and therefore our ability to digest and extract nutrients from them, is severely compromised. This is mainly because we have not had enough evolutionary time to be able to adapt to, and therefore metabolize them properly.

It is also important to note that if we have not had enough time to incorporate wheat into our diet, that sugar, which was first eaten in India and Polynesia only five hundred years ago, has a long way to go. By the way, of contemporary interest, is the fact that high fructose corn syrup used in the majority of soft drinks, as well as numerous other processed foods, has only been a regular part of the western diet since the 1970's.

If you are going to try a Paleolithic diet for your PANDAS child, remember the basics. Paleo is not the same as a high protein, low carb diet. Paleo is a diet that is high in fruit and vegetables, moderate in fat and meat intake, very low in dairy and very low in grains, with as little sugar as possible, and absolutely no corn syrup.

GAPS Diet

The Gut And Psychology Syndrome or GAPS diet, is a program based specifically on the concept that nutrition and intestinal health has a direct correlation with behavioral and learning disorders. It is similar to the gluten free diet in the sense that a leaky gut, along with the imperfect assimilation of food, is a primary cause of a number of physical and mental health problems. However, it differs in the idea that gluten is the only culprit. GAPS is also different to the Paleo diet, in that GAPS is medicinal in its focus. GAPS is a pathology specific diet, whereas Paleo is a theoretical philosophy for overall good health for everyone, regardless of their pathology.

At the heart of GAPS thinking, rests the idea that a syndrome of signs and symptoms related to psychological and physical health can all be traced back to a disturbance in the balance of intestinal microbes. There is some modern evidence to back up the claim that we truly are what we eat, or if you are a Paleo follower, we are what we have eaten. Gut bacteria has been shown to influence our moods and outlook, and consequently, GAPS interpretation says it is very important that we eat the right foods which will then promote the right gut bacteria.

I want to simplify the action of gut bacteria. Let me start with bacteria V – V for fruit and vegetables. Our body has grown used to bacteria V to such a degree, that it has developed a positive symbiotic relationship with bacteria V in just the same way as flowering plants have developed a symbiotic relationship with bees. Bacteria V lives in our body and it gives us many positive things in return. There is no such thing as unconditional love in nature. Bacteria V may not have always given us something positive and constructive, but over time our bodies have learned to absorb and use the by-products of bacteria V to such an extent that we now rely on those by-products.

However, there is something special to remember and that is that bacteria V does not live off us, otherwise it would be a harmful parasite. Bacteria V lives off the food we eat. We just beneficially synthesize the wastes and by-products that come from the digestive process provided by bacteria V. In this case, let us consider that it is our brain, or more specifically the cerebellum, that needs and utilizes the products that bacteria V provide. When bacteria V is operating at a healthy level in our gut, the more nutrients the cerebellum receives, and the more optimum it's performance.

Bacteria V is like all life; it thrives when it has the right conditions, but it is also very diet specific. Like all living creatures, bacteria V has adapted to suit its own range of foods. In this case, bacteria V loves eating fruit and vegetables. This relationship has been with us since the dawn of time and bacteria V cannot get enough. The more fruit and vegetables we eat, the more bacteria V will reproduce and excrete the beneficial elements our cerebellum needs.

However, bacteria V does not like meat and bacteria V certainly does not like refined starch. The only thing worse to bacteria V than refined starch is the bacteria Y that lives off that starch. We are going to call the bacteria necessary to digest starch - not natural starches found in whole grains, rice or potatoes, but refined starches found in white bread and sugar, pastries and donuts - bacteria Y, as in *why* bother eating it.

Refined starch may not be directly poisonous to bacteria V, but because refined starches are relatively new to our systems, bacteria V cannot utilize them. Bacteria Y is gut bacteria that can process and live off refined starches like cakes and cookies, but its wastes and by-products are not beneficial to the body, because our body has not had enough time to develop a process to effectively utilize these by-products. Waste products from bacteria V are nutrients to our body, a bit like what worm castings or compost is to our garden. The wastes from bacteria Y are just that – waste. It is equivalent to throwing bits of plastic or maybe an old TV on the garden and hoping it will nourish plants in the same way as compost.

Bacteria M – M for meat - is also in the gut, but these bacteria are more acid tolerant and live to breakdown and survive from meat. Compared to bacteria V, which has been with us forever, bacteria M is new to the evolutionary landscape. But it has been with us for three million years, so our body has learned to beneficially utilize the products that bacteria M excretes.

As you can see, we are back to Paleo philosophy and the GAPS diet, which is an extension of the 'eat clean' philosophy.

Bacteria multiply rapidly, and like all life where competition drives survival, they compete with each other. One recent study was printed in 'Livescience' 2013 and showed how volunteers were changed from a plant-based diet to a meat and dairy based diet. Gut bacteria changed significantly in type and numbers in – wait for it – one day. That's right, within twenty-four hours, the stool sample of the participants showed that the ratio of numbers between their plant eating bacteria (our bacteria V) and their more carnivorous specific bacteria (our bacteria M) had altered, with bacteria M significantly increasing in numbers. You might be tempted to say, 'so what, who cares which types of bacteria are in our gut, provided they digest the food we eat.' But it isn't all about food. It is also about the bacterial waste products. We have adapted to the by-products of bacteria M and so their waste turns into beneficial nutrients for our muscles, nervous system and our brain.

Beneficial gut bacteria also contribute to a healthy immune system by producing various anti-microbial substances. However, in order to cultivate the right gut bacteria, that is, the specific bacteria that help our body, we have to eat the food that these beneficial bacteria live off, and that's where meat, fruit, and vegetables are vital. But the majority of these bacteria survive predominantly off vegetable matter. This means a balanced meat and vegetable diet is healthy, so too is a vegetarian diet. It does not mean a meat only or a very meat heavy diet is healthy. Many researchers claim that the opposite of a carnivorous diet – a vegan diet - can also be unhealthy, particularly when it comes to by product vitamins like B12. Bottom line? Like your grandmother told you – keep it balanced.

However, the whole Paleo versus vegetarian argument of whether 'to eat meat or not to eat meat', pales into insignificance when compared to the burning question of modern times which is, what are we going to do about bacteria Y?

Processed food is filling the supermarket shelves at an ever-growing rate, about to become the main part of the family meal, for both children and overworked adults who are too tired to cook at the end of their day. The intestines and taste buds of both children and their parents are fast becoming addicted to fat, sugar, and salt. Bacteria Y is gaining a foothold and is flourishing in our systems at the cost of the beneficial compost we used to thrive on from bacteria V. The rich black compost made by bacteria V, has been replaced by the nutritional equivalent of battery acid, plastic bottles, and an old piece of carpet. Bon Appetite!

I stated early that GAPS differs from Paleo, even though both are supporters of a meat and vegies clean diet. GAPS takes its objective one-step further because GAPS is trying to be medicinal, whereas Paleo focuses on lifestyle and general health. GAPS has a specific protocol that must be followed in order to get the best results. For example, GAPS highlights the need to use meat-based soups regularly in order for the rapidly multiplying cells of the digestive tract to have all the nutrients they need for cellular repair. By keeping meat and meat products the basis of the diet, at least in the first stages, any repair to the leaks in the gut is achieved more quickly. This is also accomplished with the addition of regular doses of probiotics. Meat provides the building blocks for new cells to form, and because stomach and intestinal cells are replaced more frequently than other cells in the body, eating more meat provides more amino acids to the system, which means healthier cell reproduction and less gut leaks.

As time goes on, assorted fruits, berries, vegetables, and nuts are slowly included back into the diet. However, the GAPS diet remains, at least from a naturopathic perspective, relatively meat heavy, which does have the potential to cause an inflammatory disturbance in the bowel specifically, even if the inflammation is no longer systemic. Despite my naturopathic reservations, many of my patients' parents swear that GAPS has helped improve the behavior of their PANDAS child, at least to some degree.

Nutritional Supplements
Another aspect of treatment that may be successful is the inclusion into the daily routine of an increase in Vitamin C, Zinc, and B group vitamins, ranging in a daily dose from high to very high. Generally, I have not seen or heard via the parents of my PANDAS patients, any of the wonders that some practitioners claim using these high dose supplements. However, this could be because I am only seeing the children for whom the treatment did not work. If it did work then

they would not need to search me out, so that needs to be kept in mind in reference to what I am about to say. Mega doses of vitamins, especially individual vitamins and minerals, such as mega doses of Vitamin C, or mega doses of Zinc, are no longer a supplement, they are a medicine.

Supplemental use of vitamins is useful for a deficiency in the overall diet, with the knowledge that the addition of a certain vitamin will fill this shortfall. However, the size of the doses in mega dose therapy is way beyond any natural shortfall. In order to get ten to fifteen thousand milligrams of Vitamin C from eating oranges, you would need to sit for days on end doing nothing but peeling and eating oranges. In fact, you could never ingest that much vitamin C because your stomach would be so overburdened, you would most likely throw up half way through and have to start again.

Vitamin C is a component of many natural foods, especially fruits, but the levels demanded by many practitioners' leaves behind any idea that the vitamin is still a natural substance. This does not mean mega doses do not work; it just means this type of treatment probably should not be called natural. The same applies to mega doses of any mineral or vitamin, I am not just singling out vitamin C. That being the case, I do not want to go into this area too much, suffice to say that if this is the pathway you intend to take your PANDAS child down, please do so under professional supervision.

There are some elements to diet that are beyond dispute, but others that are very much up in the air. Is the GAPS diet better that the Paleo diet? If everything regarding PANDAS comes down to inflammation, why isn't either the vegetarian or vegan diet being mentioned, considering animal proteins are so acidic forming and inflammatory? This is a very good question. Of all the different diets parents place their PANDAS children on, vegan or vegetarian diets hardly rate a mention. This is an area unexplored but worthy of consideration.

One other very interesting aspect regarding gut bacteria is that the amount of gut bacteria we have in our body is approximately one kilogram, or just over two pounds, which is also about the size of the human brain. There are even more gut bacteria in our intestines than there are genes in the human genome. This is also an area where there is much more to learn.

So, to answer the ultimate question, does that mean my PANDAS child, or the rest of my family – parents as well – have to live a pristine lifestyle and never eat junk food or confectionary? No, and here's why. Our intestines, when it comes to gut bacteria, are just like a rainforest. Gut bacteria don't even know we exist. They just go about their normal lives like sheep in a paddock; eating, excreting, and making more sheep.

The more each type of bacteria is fed, the more that bacteria will multiply. Survival of the fittest is not just about the individual being strong and well-armed; survival of the fittest often means strength in numbers.

Plants for example, are constantly trying to out compete each other by either dropping highly acidic leaves or needles. This is so that nothing can grow underneath their canopy and therefore compete for ground nutrients or sunlight. We see this type of competition with some wattle trees, as well as pines and cyprus, while other plants try to out compete their neighbors by spreading widely and flat across the ground, prohibiting any potential competing seeds from gaining sunlight and sprouting.

The point of all this is that Bacteria V will try and out compete bacteria M and bacteria Y, while bacteria M will try and out compete bacteria V and on it goes. Every individual species of life is totally, thoroughly, and completely self-serving. Each will try their best to not only use all the available resources, but to also manipulate and change the environment so it is primarily suited to them. Not a single species will voluntarily share a thing.

However, we have something that bacteria do not have. We have the knowledge, not just the ability, to manipulate the bacteria's environment and monitor which bacteria will be dominant in our system simply by the foods we eat. But don't think for one instant that you're not being manipulated either. Have you ever noticed that the more junk food you eat, the more junk food you want to eat? Have you ever noticed that the more you get into the habit of eating something sugary and sweet after your evening meal, the more you look forward to eating something sugary straight after you finish eating? You thought this was just a bad habit of yours, a lack of willpower on your part because basically you're a weak person, right? Wrong! That's bacteria Y messing with your head.

You may have thought as you were reading about competitive plants that I was just waffling, but this information has a purpose. Gut bacteria will do their level best to out compete and change their environment so it's conducive to them and not their competitors. Here's a question for you; if bacteria Y lives off refined starches and junk food, what's the best way bacteria Y can ensure that they keep getting what they need in order to survive? Answer, by sending out chemicals that make you crave the foods they need to survive.

Bacteria are evolutionary speedsters, they can adapt and share information at a rate that is so far beyond human beings it's not funny. Antibiotic resistant bacteria are a perfect example of this. Bacteria V probably used to make us crave veggies a long time ago, but over time it has become so integrated with our system that our health reliance has been enough of a stimulus for us to keep eating them. But glowing health is not the by-product of bacteria Y, in fact it is the opposite. So if bacteria Y is going to survive – and no life form ever wants to just lay down and die – then it has to come up with another strategy to make us eat what it requires. And it has worked out the perfect way. After releasing its own waste, that same waste triggers a part of our brain to create in us the desire to eat more of the food that bacteria Y relies on.

Isn't that just a symbiotic relationship, the same as we have with bacteria V you might ask? No. We are healthier because of bacteria V. We thrive off them just as much as they thrive off us. We not only get little or next to nothing regarding health benefits from bacteria Y, but their wastes are acidic and poisonous to our system. For every bit of energy we may get from consuming foods compatible with bacteria

Y, we spend ten bits of energy processing, detoxing, and repairing the damage that bacteria has done.

If you have a PANDAS child and their energy to symptoms balance is precarious at the best of times, they don't need foods that feed bacteria Y. In fact, for kids with PANDAS, or indeed anybody at all, we have to move away from labeling these products as foods at all. There used to be an old saying back in the middle ages regarding syphilis and how the disease was contracted. The saying went 'A night with Venus and a lifetime with Mercury,' Venus being the goddess of love and the element mercury being the cure at that time for the disease. I admit this saying is perhaps a little over the top when it comes to PANDAS and junk food, but the minute of enjoyment your PANDAS child may get by giving them a sugary treat is not worth the hours and hours of hell that follows for you as the parent. Until their system is back in balance and they are able to digest and tolerate these treats without complications, you have to ask yourself, is giving them this treat worth it? If not, Y bother.

The other thing to keep in mind when dealing with diet and PANDAS is that the waste by-products of bacteria Y don't just stimulate us to crave more junk food. I believe they also directly influence our behavior and emotions. And this is not confined to just bacteria Y, but includes bacteria V and M as well. The following hypothesis is not PANDAS specific, but it's an interesting concept nonetheless.

I have an idea that not only do these gut bacteria make us crave what they need to survive, but I am going to take this concept even further by proposing that it's a distinct possibility that specific colonies of gut bacteria create an environment, via the nutritional triggers of their by-products, that makes us physically and mentally better equipped to have the skills necessary to satisfy these cravings.

If you take bacteria M for example, not only will it create a desire for fat and meat, but synthesized meat will provide amino acids and vitamins like vitamin B12, which cannot be obtained from any other unfortified plant source. Vitamin B12 is vital for both red blood cells as well as for the central nervous system.

Now think of what skills you need for hunting; coordinated and rapid muscle control, and enough oxygen to maintain an extended level of strength and endurance. These functions simply could not be achieved without vitamin B12.

Now here is the circle unbroken. We started eating meat, which meant we needed gut bacteria specific for the task of breaking the meat down. However, because gut bacteria are organic life forms, they are going to eat, excrete, move, and multiply. Instead of being poisoned by their waste products, human beings have learned to utilize and capitalize the waste from bacteria M and turn it into something beneficial. In fact, it is now something so beneficial, that we to rely on these nutrients to survive. The nutrients supplied by meat, and the by-products of the bacteria M cycle, are now used by the body to make us more successful hunters. This in turn increases our chances of catching more meat, which is mutually beneficial to both us and bacteria M.

However, I'm not sure the symbiotic relationship between humans and gut bacteria ends there. Certain mental and emotional traits are also needed in order to be a successful hunter. For example, the hunter's senses must be extremely acute and their nervous system must be highly reactive. It is quite likely that people whose intestines are dominant in bacteria M will display these highly acute senses and reactive nervous systems. They may even be more aggressive because this is the required food cycle. You need strength, aggression, and reactivity, if you are going to be a good hunter. The areas of the body that provide these traits rely on a constant supply of the type of nutrients provided by meat and the by-products of the bacteria that digest meat. Our gut is an ecosystem and like all thriving ecosystems, it works on a strong co-dependent reliance.

On the other side of the coin, let's take a look at what is needed to be a good gatherer or forager. First of all, you need persistence, accuracy, stamina, and concentration. After all, in the forest, sometimes the berries or leaves of a poisonous plant can closely resemble the edible berries you want to pick for dinner. You must be accurate or the consequences could be dire.

So here's the thing if we want to be smart. The brain may not be the biggest organ in the body, but it's certainly the greediest when it comes to munching down on kilojoules or calories. In fact, between a fifth to a quarter of all our kilojoules are utilized by the brain. However, and this is an important however, the brain only eats these kilojoules in the form of glucose and some fat.

Glucose is brain food, and the best way to keep the brain bathed in the constant supply of glucose it requires, is to graze rather than gobble down food, and to eat foods with a slow but constant glucose release. In modern times these foods are called low GI foods; in the olden days it was called healthy eating. The foods that supply the glucose requirements in the form our brain requires are fruits and vegetables. They are the perfect gatherer food for the hunter-gatherer lifestyle and most have a low GI index. The type of fat the brain likes, which is mainly omega 3, can be sourced through nuts and seeds.

In order to survive, we need to know what plants we can eat and what plants we can't, and in order to know that, we have to be smart. We have to remember and be able to identify which plants taste good and which plants do us harm, and we not only have to remember these details, we have to be able to pass this knowledge on to the next generation otherwise trial and error starts all over again. Bacteria V and the nutrition from plants fires our brain, which makes us smart so we can identify and cook the plants that will help make us and bacteria V thrive.

Meat eating bacteria give us nutrients that in turn, give us the ability to react to our surroundings. Plant eating bacteria give us the clarity to process what these now heightened senses take in. This is great news for people with intestines filled with bacteria M and bacteria V, but what about a person whose gut is high in bacteria Y?

The easiest way to understand what kind of emotional temperament will be produced after eating a particular food, is to look at what skills are needed to acquire that type of food in the first place. Strength and sharp senses are needed for hunting, so in return eating meat heightens our muscular strength and our senses. Gathering requires knowledge and endurance, and in return these foods bathe our brain with glucose and supply our bodies with a low GI food source.

But what about that soda drink you have in your hand, or the chocolate bar you are just about to eat, or perhaps that packet of macaroni and cheese you just had for dinner? What skills did you need to acquire it? That's right – none. You opened the packet because you were tired, or you don't like to cook, or because you felt lazy. The personality that develops from bacteria Y is equal to the intent of why you chose it in the first place. Lazy breeds lazy, and I don't care, breeds I don't care. Why do you eat too much chocolate? Because it is yummy and gives instant gratification, the same as all sweets.

So we are we surprised when a child full of bacteria Y screams dissatisfaction? Bacteria Y foods aren't hunted or gathered, they are given to you easily, quickly and conveniently, so it should be no surprise that people dominated by bacteria Y will lack will power, endurance, and yet be expectant.

PANDAS kids and bacteria Y is a toxic combination - socially, physically, and mentally. DO NOT MIX!! As a parent reading this you must understand that this is not a health warning for the future. If your PANDAS child gets too much packet food and sweets in their diet, the ramifications are immediate and dire. You are not giving your PANDAS child a treat by giving in to their junk food demands – it is not an act of kindness, and they will not thank you for it. In fact, I can tell you now that you will never have a good relationship with your PANDAS child because their system is going crazy under the stress of this 'food', and in this state, the world and everyone in it becomes their enemy.

There is an interesting process and intent behind the history of sugar and junk food.

Hunters and gatherers saw the forest as a nurturing and loving mother who provided for our needs. Many indigenous tribes would thank the gods for the animals that died so the tribe could eat. Sugar came into prominence out of colonialism, conquest, and the misery of slavery, while junk food developed as a cheap way to fill the stomachs of those who don't want to cook, or can't afford too much - but you always get what you pay for.

12

PANDAS AND EXERCISE

This exercise chapter will be much smaller than the chapter on diet because exercise it is less complicated overall - at least for PANDAS kids. As a general principle, there is no need to discuss common exercise topics of debate such as: is cardio training more effective for weight loss than weight training, or how many times a week should I exercise in order to get the best effects without wasting energy, or even how should I vary my exercise routine? These are all adult exercise questions, so they don't have much of a place for children.

The bottom line for exercise and PANDAS kids is pretty simple – allow them as much as they need and whatever movement they enjoy. Note here that I did not say for them to do as much exercise as they want, because as many PANDAS parents already know, their PANDAS child's need for exercise and their desire to do exercise can be two different things entirely. Some PANDAS kids will run all day if you let them. Their nervous system seems to be boundless when it comes to energy, which can be either a good or a bad thing, depending on whether their energy is focused or scattered. Most hyperactive kids, while bursting with energy, are not bursting with focused or usable energy. In fact, focused energy seems to be in short supply. Most of the time, the energy surging inside a lot of PANDAS kids is spent fiddling, scratching, wriggling and squirming, jumping up and down, or running from place to place, or from activity to activity, rarely, if ever, achieving anything.

This is what I mean when I refer to energy as being scattered, unfocused, or unusable. Focused energy is the best kind of energy, but so few PANDAS kids seem to have it. Anxiety or obsessional OCD is not focused energy, despite the amount of effort that seems to go into keeping these habits alive. Scattered PANDAS energy is not productive and can inhibit them intellectually, physically, or socially.

PANDAS is a hydra-headed syndrome, so some children display no hyperactivity at all. Other PANDAS kids are very capable of focusing their energy, so for them the ability to stick to an allotted task is no problem at all. They are able to focus for extended periods of time and then do as much exercise as they can handle. For these kids, the PANDAS symptoms center on tics, repeating words or phrases, or perhaps in some worrying thoughts or fears that just won't leave them. Wherever your child falls on the spectrum, it is still a good idea to include exercise as part of their daily or weekly routine, simply because exercise settles the nervous system and a settled nervous system is vital for a PANDAS child's stability.

For many PANDAS kids however, the topic of exercise can be a volatile one. Commonly these kids complain about their difficulties in getting to, or staying asleep – often a direct result of too little exercise in a young body. Often PANDAS kids display other associated symptoms that demonstrate they are not getting enough exercise.

It can be a touchy subject, simply because many PANDAS kids feel so insecure about themselves. Many also have poor motor co-ordination and therefore lack the sporting skills that would make them feel physically successful. As a flow on effect, their insecurities begin to turn into reality, as their lack of co-ordination or their lack of focus makes them far from the star player on the team. Despite parental reassurances that they don't have to be a star to enjoy playing the game, or that the purpose of sport is to go out and have a good time, the feeling of being less capable than others leaves some PANDAS kids skeptical of sport being fun. Many are aware that their athletic skill level is deficient by comparison to others, and this can add extra pressure as they feel the need to be even better than average in order to compensate for their shortcomings. So they make the decision that if they can't be extra good, they won't do that sport at all. Many of these kids will go to where most struggling kids in the modern age go – to the world where they are in control and the place where real skills won't be tested - video games.

A lot of parents may think, 'So, what's wrong with that? Video games are creative and besides, kids like them and all their friends are doing it?' But for a PANDAS child there are so many things wrong with video games it's difficult to know where to begin.

First and foremost, playing a video game is not exercise. There may be a lot of characters running around on the screen with explosions going off everywhere, but the kid with the controller munching down their snacks ain't movin' that's for sure! And no, twiddling thumbs and pushing buttons is not regarded as aerobic exercise. No matter how many ninjas' your child may fight, their muscle tone will not improve.

However, one thing that will increase as your PANDAS child becomes more and more immersed into their video games is their anger and intolerance at being disturbed, and this occurs for two reasons. First, their natural OCD tendency changes form and switches from fear and specific daily rituals into a total absorption and preoccupation with the game they are playing. Does it replace their tics, fears, or routines? No, in fact, video games intensify these problems. It is just that for some kids, their tics or fears can be put on hold while their mind is absorbed in the game. While they are immersed in this electronic place life is easy and life is good but when the time comes to bring them back - watch out - because the person who is trying to reach in and grab them is going to incur their full wrath, and in a PANDAS child that wrath can be untempered.

The type of exercise PANDAS kids (and all kids) need is 'organic' exercise. That is, exercise that has a natural base and focus. There may be props involved but they are the old fashioned variety; balls, bats, goal posts, bikes and even kites. Obviously weather or supervision may be a factor, but outside exercise is the best form for children. Fresh air has considerable positive outcomes because fresh air revitalizes the body energetically.

Movement and the deep breathing of fresh air go hand in hand. They are the duo of good energy. But there is a third factor that is often forgotten. When kids play outside with balls and bikes they are often with other kids and playing (exercising) with other kids is fun. Fun is a huge energy regenerator. Laughing and moving and breathing in fresh air will help your PANDAS child immensely.

In this day and age, we are so focused on safety, we often forget that these moments outside with other children (with few or no boundaries) shape a child's view of the world and build a confidence and curiosity that provides a platform they will carry into adulthood. Video games are a poor and even debilitating substitute.

Case 6
Liam – male aged 10
When Liam first became a patient, he was in a pretty bad emotional and nervous state. Even though his mother was loving and smart, her available time was fractured and her knowledge regarding nutrition was limited. Even what she thought she knew regarding nutrition needed - well let's just say, there were some rough edges that needed smoothing over. Do I think this is her fault? Absolutely not. Modern life is full of double think and it's almost impossible for most people to know the difference between the truth, the ownership of the truth, and the marketing of truth. Ninety percent of the population is passive when it comes to most daily topics. Some know all about nutrition but are passively compliant when it comes to car maintenance. They just accept what their mechanic tells them needs to be done to their car and hope they can trust their honesty. Everyone is ten percent active and ninety percent passive. Liam's mum was passively knowledgeable about nutrition. The trouble is, can you trust your source?

Let's take a simple example. Everyone knows soup is great to eat when you're sick, right? Why? Because soup is virtually predigested, so the amount of energy your body needs to expend metabolizing the ingredients is negligible by comparison to eating those same foods whole. This means, if we are talking about pumpkin soup for example, that the energy used by the body will be less than the energy normally used to process the pumpkin if it was cooked and served as a vegetable on a plate. Also, any nutrients that are leaked from the vegetable during the cooking process go directly into the water that makes up the soup, rather than being lost.

But are all soups the same? Is a can of pumpkin soup with its history of food processing the same as a homemade soup eaten straight after it is cooked? For so many reasons the answer is no. When a soup manufacturer tells you that nutritional science gives the tick of approval to their soup as a nourishing food, they are making you associate those nutritional facts to the product they want you to buy. But the product on the shelf is often much older soup than the soup used in the nutritional study. This makes the truth, and what you think is the truth, two different concepts. One is the truth, the other is the marketing of the truth.

Science often talks about the calorific value of food (in energetic terms) and it talks about the nutritional content of food, but do you ever hear science talk about the importance of the life force of food? Of course not, and the reason is simple. Medical science does not believe in anything that cannot be measured, or if you want to be even more skeptical, some might say that medical science does not believe in any concept that does not fit into the medical science paradigm of thinking. So when naturopaths talk about the energy of food, they are not just referring to calories or kilojoules, but also to the life force inside the food.

Life force has a spiritual quality. It is the unseen force that brings a baby to life and continues to make it grow and develop without any conscious thought or participation from the parents, outside of the conception itself of course. Life force is what makes cells divide and people both conscious and animated. Life force is in everything organic and as $E=MC^2$ has proven, it is also in everything inorganic as well. Even though it is commonly accepted that there are enormous amounts of energy packed inside every speck of matter, what does medical science say when an alternative therapist talks about concepts like life force or life energy? They say it's unscientific, unprovable, hippie rubbish because they have no pills or treatment, and therefore no way of utilizing this energy, even if they were to concede it was real. That's the difference between the truth, and the ownership of the truth.

Life force does exist. But if that truth was accepted it would also mean that any medical system that does not cater for this energy must, by definition, be incomplete and deficient. So scientific medicine accepts that energy is real and present, but only in atoms (despite the fact that we are nothing but atoms) and that energy can only to be used by technology, but not by people. Historically this sounds very much like how the divide between science and the church was originally solved. Both agreed that humans did have a soul, but then they compromised by saying that the soul was separate to the physical body. That meant medicine could have the body to work on, while the church still had dominion over our eternal wellbeing. Now the divide has switched its focus. Yes, there is an internal energy, but that energy only exists inside things that we don't treat as patients. Atoms may vibrate with an inner resonant energy, but collections of atoms like human beings and animals do not - now that's selective science.

That is a long winded answer to why I didn't blame Liam's mother for being confused about the rights and wrongs of nutrition, lifestyle, and exercise. The good thing was that it didn't take long for her to understand that packaged food and jars of sauce do not have the same quality and goodness as home-made food. To her credit she persisted, in fact the only person more tenacious than Liam in his refusal to eat good food, was his mother and her own tenacity to make sure he did. Eventually she got smart and started hiding vegetables in sauces she knew Liam would eat. To cut a long story short, his diet became pretty good.

Liam had a likable nature. He was curious, involved, and social. His problem was his excessive nervous anxiety and his physical tics. His anxiety displayed itself most typically as night time fears and rituals. His fears were changeable. One night they would be ghosts or monsters, the next it would be storms. If the weather report was clear then his anxiety would switch to robbers or kidnappers. He was also afraid that he had done something wrong, even when there was no reason.

I have treated many PANDAS kids who have a 'wrong' anxiety but after treating patient after patient with PANDAS, I know that their sense of wrong can be very individualized. Making a mistake or being wrong for some PANDAS kids means they think they are not a good person, and they want to be a good person, therefore they can never be wrong. For others, wrong takes on a more spiritual meaning, and they can be in anguish over the state of their soul and whether they are good enough for heaven, or because they occasionally think bad thoughts, they live in fear that they are going to hell. Another form of 'wrong' belongs to those PANDAS kids who constantly feel that they have offended someone. At night, these kids will agonize over the events of their day, searching to free themselves of the burden that someone is upset with them over a callous statement, or an action they may have performed.

Liam belonged to the second category of fear. He would have violent thoughts like 'what would happen if I threw a knife at this person?' Or 'what would happen if I punched him or her really hard in the face?' Liam was not a violent kid and he knew he would never act on his thoughts. In fact, he was so appalled by his own private thoughts that he started believing he should not leave the house.

The tics Liam experienced were head rolling, a stomping action, and dragging his right foot on the ground in the manner one would expect to see from an agitated horse.

Liam's main ambition was to play baseball. He loved baseball, although I forget the name of the team he was passionate about. His mum, for what she called selfish motives, wanted Liam to become enthusiastic and play for a basketball team. Her reasoning was sound. Basketball is interesting, and it only lasts forty minutes. Baseball is slow and can drag on for three or four hours. In Australia we play cricket not baseball, and the same game of cricket can last for five days! She got no sympathy from me.

Liam's desire to play baseball was a trump card I often don't get to play. For a lot of PANDAS kids, getting them to follow what I would like them to do is often a difficult task. Many PANDAS kids refuse point blank to eat anything I suggest, or to do any exercise, no matter how much I try and coerce them.

Thankfully, most of the time it's not me who has to try and convince them, it's their parents. I have had many successful PANDAS cases with kids I have never even met. A lot of PANDAS kids are way too sensitive about their thoughts and feelings to ever blurt them out to another person other than their mum or dad, but that's okay. Luckily I can do most cases based on the information provided by one or both of the parents. In cases where the child won't help themselves by making any positive changes to their diet or lifestyle, everything comes down to the remedy I select. I can still get through and make vital changes to PANDAS kids who refuse to comply, but where good eating and exercise are introduced, progress is much faster.

With Liam however, the case was different. The carrot of baseball was so tempting he was ready to try anything that would help him get out on to the field. So he accepted the changes his mother put in place, and when I asked him to help walk the dog every night, because regular exercise would help his nervous system, Liam, unlike most PANDAS kids, agreed. These actions, together with the well-chosen remedy, saw Liam improve quickly and dramatically.

In the first month after treatment, Liam went from sleeping on the floor in his mother's room every night – which I didn't even know until our follow up consultation – to sleeping in his own bed.

By the second follow up two months later, Liam was still in his own bed, but also falling asleep early, because he was not worried about thoughts so much. His violent thoughts were still occurring, but now they were fleeting rather than ever present and demanding. Two months after treatment, Liam felt that he was in control of his thoughts rather than the other way around.

By the third follow up, Liam's head rolling tic had all but disappeared. His leg tic had also diminished considerably.

By the fourth follow up Liam felt confident enough to join a school T-Ball team. I'm not sure what that is exactly but Liam was ecstatic, because he believed he was on the way to realizing his baseball dream.

By the fifth follow up, which was now at two monthly intervals rather than one month because Liam was improving so well, his intrusive thoughts were rare. In his own words, he was only having them once every few weeks, if that. Liam told me that his tics were completely gone, although his mother said afterwards that was not quite true. However, they were lessened to such a degree that they were only noticeable to her. They were mother's tics; slight little twitches observable to her, but to everyone else, including Liam, they couldn't be seen.

I see no reason whatsoever why Liam won't be playing baseball next year. If I didn't live on the other side of the globe, I would go and watch him play.

For Homeopaths
The rubrics I chose to repertorise included –

> MIND; FEAR; night (84)
> MIND; VIOLENCE, vehemence (124)
> HEAD; MOTIONS; of, shaking, nodding, waving (122)
> EXTREMITIES; MOTIONS (144)

One of the things to take notice of in this repertorisation is the rubric 'Violence' rather than the rubric 'Thoughts, violent'. The reason for this is because the thoughts of violence rubric only had one remedy and that narrows down my choices considerably! I do not like small rubrics when repertorising, but I can understand why practitioners who have no other way of discriminating between remedies use them. For me, it's a different story. Facial analysis means I only select remedies that have the same inherent force as my patient, so my repertorisation can be broad and based solely on what is observable and known.

Leaving out subjective interpretation of symptoms makes for great accuracy. That being said, occasionally an interpretation is necessary, as can be seen in the rubric violence. Normally this rubric would literally mean an act of violence or a violent person rather than a placid person having violent thoughts. But with only one remedy under 'Thoughts violent' I was left with no other option than to think laterally. To the question, 'Why don't I give the remedy that is under the rubric 'Thoughts violent'? My answer; because a single rubric does not represent the totality of symptoms and the totality of symptoms is the foundation of the similimum. When a homeopath is trying to find the similimum, they are like an artist reproducing a portrait of the patient. Repertorisation belongs to the realm of realism, not surrealism, and definitely not cubism.

Liam's facial analysis showed that he belonged to the blue (syphilitic) group. This means his system will defend itself by conserving energy when it is under stress. Two blue remedies had every rubric in Liam's repertorisation – Aurum Metallicum and Mercury. Aurum was chosen as the first choice, simply because it was numerically higher than Mercury. Aurum was so successful that no remedy change was required. Aurum was given in the 30C potency once daily.

13

OBSESSIONS AND OCD

An obsession is like a passion, except an obsession has no lingering feeling of fulfillment, so there is no sense of achievement or reward at the end. An obsession, like an addiction, is a cycle of net loss. You need to keep getting more and more of the 'fix', or a stronger and stronger 'hit', just to achieve the same reward. A seekers passion for knowledge, or a mother's passion for her family, gives meaning to life and a reason to exist. OCD has that same intense drive and that same burning desire, except that with OCD in general and almost always when part of the PANDAS picture, there is no feeling of success and no sense of accomplishment. So there is no satisfaction and no satiety. That means the yearning hole is never filled. All that is left is more yearning.

PANDAS kids often find a way to focus their susceptibility for OCD, and it is not usually in a healthy way. Video games are a great example, and what is especially bad about this type of past-time, is that most video games are designed for stimulation and excitement. If they were dull, no one would play them. The trouble with PANDAS and too much excitement is that stimulation shoots adrenalin throughout the system, and a body full of adrenalin is the last thing a typical PANDAS child needs.

Most PANDAS kids, although not all, already live in a state of fight or flight. I don't know why this mechanism is switched on so permanently, but for many PANDAS children it is and that's what the family and the practitioner have to work with. The behaviors that manifest as part of the syndrome can be time consuming and part of an overall paranoid picture. These fight or flight kids can check under their bed and in their cupboards for villains who may have broken into the house and who are waiting to get them on a nightly basis. Parents waste countless hours checking and re-checking potential hiding places, just so their child can finally go to sleep. As a PANDAS child gets older, they may confess to their parents that they don't really believe a robber is in the house – but just to be sure could they check anyway.

This type of PANDAS child has numerous fears, not just of robbers and kidnappers. They might be afraid of heights, of insects, dogs, traffic, or strangers. They might be afraid of germs, of being wrong, of what other people are thinking, or of being discovered that they are not a good person because of the bad thoughts they are experiencing. These examples are all common PANDAS thoughts, and fortunately they are frequently removed, or at the very least dramatically modified, during subsequent treatment.

As a result of this fight or flight mental state, the body responds with either hyperactivity and fruitless restlessness, or a state of internal muscular or nervous tension. So what does this mean in relation to playing video games?

If a child's constitution is already in a state of high alert, the last thing they need is more excitement in their system. That's where a knowledge of what happens when playing video games becomes important, because excitation is what most of these games are designed to produce. Your PANDAS child will scoff at the suggestion that video games are in any way unhealthy, but then most PANDAS kids are obsessed with video games, so they will defend them in any way they can. Many will argue that they are old enough to know the difference between reality and a video game, after all they're not an idiot, but video games are an area where imagination and reality can start to blur a little, and that means life can become a little tricky.

In order to grasp this understanding, it's important to remember that there is a vast difference between conscious awareness and instinctive muscle memory. Your truth may not be your body's truth, and your understanding may not be your body's understanding.

Here's a fact; everyone knows that an on screen drama is not real life, right? Okay, then I have a question, why do you jump in a scary movie, and why does your heart race during a stressful scene? Why does your body start to tense up and sweat, as the actor's arm searching for something down a drain, comes perilously close to a rearing snake, or a disease-ridden rat? Look at the patrons of the theatre during the next romance movie you see (apart from a lot of the husbands who have been dragged along against their will) and witness as the screen husband holds the hand of his young dying wife, breathing her last breath and whispering to him to look after the children with her last 'I love you.' There won't be a dry eye in the house and yet everyone in the cinema knows it's a movie. We know it's a script. We know these people are actors and we know it's not real life, and yet your body, depending on the movie, is weeping, sweating, tense, or happy, irrespective of the fact that we know it's not real.

This concept has been written about in many journals and books; your mind is not your brain. Your brain uses your senses to analyze information about the outside world. It then conveys those impressions to the rest of the body, so the body can be in harmony, and in readiness, to respond to what the brain concludes is happening in the environment.

The thug on the screen will play havoc with your brain, which then relays those concerns to the body. Seeing the thug on screen and witnessing their sardonic smile, will make your nervous system go into a state of stress, but do you ever really believe that the exact same actor is waiting with evil intentions inside your bedroom cupboard?

Conscious awareness and instinctive physical response are not the same thing and they are not always in harmony. This disconnect is what lies beneath many acquired chronic diseases. Anyone – nothing to do with PANDAS at the moment, this is yet another digression – can go through a stressful and torrid event in their life. It may be a single event, or it may be a series of stressful events. A few years later that same person starts to develop symptoms of chronic disease. This chronic disease could be either mental or emotional, like depression or panic attacks, or it could be physical, like arthritis or cancer. The disease could be anything at all, and as surprising as this may sound, the diagnosis can often be secondary to understanding the stress that preceded it.

Scientific medicine denounces this concept. To science, understanding the person instead of understanding the disease is nonsense. But focusing only on the disease and ignoring the person who has it, as well as the stress that came before the disease, is faulty logic. The medical philosophy that disease pathology is all that matters is grossly incomplete. I'm not saying that it's ineffective when it comes to relieving pain or treating a specific pathology, just that it's an unfinished system in regards to restoring vitality and health. Many practitioners, both conventional and alternate, say that these two medical systems contradict one another and therefore can't be used in tandem, but that's not true. I have treated large numbers of patients who have also been under the care of their doctor and on conventional medications, but still got a positive outcome.

I have also had patients who will agree with the conscious awareness versus instinctive memory philosophy, but then swear black and blue that this is not why they have a chronic illness. They have had therapy for their stress, and now their head is in a completely different place to where it was when the stress first took place. Their physical ailment or their physical suffering cannot possibly be as a consequence of that prior stress.

Psychological therapies play an invaluable role in modern society, but I must stress that it needs to be understood that there is a big difference between awareness and instinctive muscle memory. Psychological therapies talk directly to our conscious understanding, but not to our survival instinct. Just because you have a different view on life now, doesn't mean your body has forgotten the danger or the stress of the past. Counsellors talk to the mind, they do not exchange ideas with the liver, lungs, or bones. This is where a well-chosen homeopathic remedy has a special place.

Back to PANDAS and video games. Just like movies, games are designed to elicit a specific emotional response. By directly influencing our emotions, entertainment in the form of stories, movies, and games, breach the outer logical conscious barrier to strike at the heart of limbic reaction. Awareness or consciousness is separate from the body. It is not a by-product of the brain, and there is no evidence to suggest that consciousness even lives in the brain. Clearly if the brain has been damaged, consciousness is effected, but that doesn't prove that consciousness comes from the brain. Just that consciousness needs some aspects of the brain to be in good working order for consciousness to able to express itself out into the world. You can have an idea without your body responding, but you can't have an emotion without your body responding.

Emotions belong to the brain, not to awareness, and the brain must keep the body in harmony. The brain is built on a three musketeers system – all for one and one for all. When you feel happy, your liver, lungs, and bones feel happy. When you feel sad, your liver, lungs and bones feel sad. The brain makes sure you are a coordinated system, that's its job.

One research study regarding muscle response trialed at Bishop's University Canada (Shackell and Standing – Mind Over Matter: Mental Training Increases Physical Strength), tested weight training gains made by three distinct groups. Group one lifted no weights and did little if anything outside of their daily routine. Group two focused on strengthening a specific muscle by repeating the same weight routine. That way monitoring any gains or changes would be easier than performing a varied routine. Group three did no actual weight lifting at all, instead they listened to a guided tape that imaginatively walked them through the step by step process of performing certain weight training exercises.

At the end of the experiment group one – the ones who didn't do anything, showed no muscle strength gains. Group two – the ones who did actual weight training - saw on average a 28% improvement in strength gains, while group three – the group who imaginatively trained – made strength gains of 24%. Almost as good as the actual training group except that group three didn't lift a finger. Adds a new dimension to 'all in the mind' doesn't it?

In one Harvard study, a group of housekeepers were all told that what they did for a living should be categorized as physical exercise. One month after being told that their daily routine was not just work but equal to a daily workout, every single one of the group had lost weight despite the fact that none of them had changed their out of work exercise routine or their diet in any way.

The brain is complex but the brain is not smart. Awareness is smart but it is separate from the body. The two come together to form a complex human being.

PANDAS kids have nervous systems that are already too impressionable and they have emotions that are already too labile. These children will be greatly affected by games that alter their emotions.

At the same time as highlighting all this electronic negativity, I realize that socially, video games are important because nearly every other kid in the first world is playing them, especially boys, so cutting your PANDAS child off from games could affect them socially. So for many parents, the key to video games is management rather than prohibition, and this is where exercise becomes vital. For every half an hour playing videos, there should be a fifteen-minute exercise program just to burn off the stress.

PANDAS kids are highly impressionable, so they will finish their game hyped up and excited. Make exercise a pre-condition to playing their game. They will never agree to exercise while they are buzzing, so make sure they understand what they have to do after the game, before they even begin to play. The type of exercise is irrelevant just as long as they burn off their excess energy so their nervous system can return to normalcy. Hyped up PANDAS kids will often refuse to calm down because their heightened state is more exciting that normal boring life. This means that in the beginning, no matter how much they promise to go outside later, or to take the dog for a walk, or ride their bike, they are most probably not going to do it without a fight, until a routine is established. As a parent, you need to stick to your guns and not give in on this one because you will both pay the price if there is no discipline or release associated with these games.

In the adult world, we choose our exercise experiences based on what we want to achieve. If we want to be fitter and keep up with our friends without panting like an old dog, then cardio training is our choice. If we want to be buff and feel strong and confident, then weights may be more suitable. Some people don't want either. They want to feel supple and free, so flexibility training or yoga is their choice. With PANDAS kids, exercise is about burning off energy and re-settling the nervous system back into a state of calm. Any exercise will physically do that, but they also have to do something they love doing in order to get their mind away from the game they just played. So whether it's playing on swings and monkey bars, or playing an organized sport, changing the emotions set in place by the game is of primary importance.

14

FINDING OUT ABOUT HOMEOPATHY

I have been clinically using homeopathy for almost a quarter of a century, which probably sounds reassuring to you, but amazing and a little bit scary for me. Where did that time go?

What I am about to do is to give you a completely one eyed and biased opinion regarding this topic, simply because this systems' counter claimers have all the money, and therefore all the press, to get their just as biased opinions across.

For every positive claim about homeopathy, there are nineteen counter claimers ready to voice their opinion. Most of these 'opinions' aren't really coming from people at all, instead they are coming from robots; programs designed to search the net looking for specific words, like acupuncture or homeopathy, to which they then post their already written out scripts. I used to wonder how and why all these negative people could search out, or even want to search out, every alternative medicinal claim, just so they could post their 'voice of reason' and their poorly disguised 'balanced' argument. I started thinking that being a skeptic must be a full time job. Then someone I know, far more advanced in the area of computer technology than I could ever be, looked at me quizzically as if surely the penny should have dropped by now, and alerted me to the fact that most of these 'people' were programs; suddenly it all made sense. No wonder they were so quick on the draw.

The odds are stacked against anything medically alternative. I do not know how many times I have heard other very credible professionally trained homeopaths say how they have tried to add their point of view to sites like Wikipedia, only to have their posts denied or changed immediately. Nearly every sentence on the homeopathy wiki pages is negative and draws conclusions and makes negative statements, instead of just presenting the facts. But then again Jimmy Wales, the founder of Wikipedia, is also on record as saying that holistic medicine is the 'work of lunatic charlatans.'

Next time you are looking at Wikipedia have a look at the references at the bottom of the homeopathy page. Hardly a homeopathic opinion in sight. Nearly every reference is a conventional medical viewpoint. If I wanted to look up a subject I would like to hear from people who have been trained and work at the coal face of the area, not from someone who tells me what they think I should believe - and has a financial interest in denying any efficacy. But that's exactly what you're getting because Wikipedia's right to free speech and knowledge only extends to what they decide you should know.

It seems we are back to the ownership of truth again. Asking conventional medical sources to be almost the sole contributor to an article on homeopathy, is like asking Donald Trump to write an article titled 'Why America should become a communist state'.

If you read about homeopathy on Wikipedia, there is a lot of information left out. For example, how the Indian government has a ministry specifically dedicated to yoga, Ayurveda medicine, naturopathy and homeopathy because the promotion and advancement of health of its people is vital for the country's future. And how these alternative medical systems are a cost effective and efficient way of achieving that aim. According to the World Health Organization's medical officer for traditional medicines, Dr. X Zhang, homeopathy has been successfully integrated into the medical systems of Germany, Mexico, Sri Lanka and the United Kingdom. But these facts don't make it to Wikipedia. And there are many other countries which also have homeopathy built into their health systems from South and Central America, to Europe, as well as India.

What about the meta-analysis of 89 trials of homeopathic medicine versus placebo, published in the Lancet 1998, that showed significantly in favor of homeopathy? (Volume 350, No. 9081, p8334-843, 20 September 1997). What about the survey of over 900 patients treated homeopathically, who showed substantial improvement in their quality of life over the first six months after treatment, and this effect remained more or less stable over the following years?

This last survey was published by The European Network of Homeopathic Researchers in 2005. I know some might scream bias, but if that is the case, we should also stop pharmaceutical manufacturers conducting trials on their own products. One of the things I learned quickly after entering alternative medicine, is that claims of bias and conclusions of placebo only flow one way.

I want to highlight some positive results from the European Network of Homeopathic Researchers as quoted above.

> *A study of 829 patients treated with homeopathic medicines, where conventional treatment had been unsatisfactory or contraindicated, concluded that 61% had a substantial improvement with homeopathy.*
>
> *A meta-analysis of 105 trials with interpretable results, 81 of those trials showed positive results for homeopathy. Most studies showed results in favour of homeopathy, even among those randomized controlled trials that received high- quality ratings for randomization, blinding, sample size, and other methodological criteria.*
>
> *HMRG reported with overview of clinical research in homeopathy, identified 184 controlled clinical trials. They selected the highest quality randomized control trials, which included a total of 2617 patients for a meta-analysis. This meta-analysis resulted in a p-value of 0.000036 (which means that results are highly significant), indicating that homeopathy is*

more effective than placebo. The researchers concluded that the "hypothesis "that homeopathy has no effect, can be rejected with certainty"

Treatment of acute childhood diarrhoea in Nicaragua. This trial involved 81 children aged from 6 months to 5 years in a randomised, double-blind trial of intravenous fluids, plus placebo versus intravenous fluids, plus a homeopathic remedy individualised to the patient. The treatment group had a statistically significant decrease in duration of diarrhoea.

Homeopathy versus conventional treatment in respiratory tract complaints. In an outcome study, 30 practitioners in four countries enrolled 500 consecutive patients, with at least one of three complaints: upper respiratory tract complaints including allergies; lower respiratory tract complaints including allergies; or ear complaints. Of 456 patients, 281 received homeopathy and 175 conventional treatment. The primary outcomes criterion was response to treatment, defined as cured or major improvement after 14 days of treatment. Results showed a response rate of 82.6% in the homeopathy group compared to 67.3% in the group receiving conventional medicine. The authors concluded that homeopathy appeared to be at least as effective as the conventional treatment of patients, with the three conditions studied.

Osteoarthritis. In this trial, 65 sufferers of Osteoarthritis (OA), were split into 2 groups, and through a double blinding process were given either a homoeopathic medicine or Acetaminophen, a commonly prescribed drug for pain relief in OA. Researchers found that homoeopathy provided a level of pain relief that was superior to Acetaminophen, and produced no adverse reactions.

Homeopathy in menopausal complaints. In a prospective study, 82 % of 102 patients, reported improvement of menopause symptoms after homeopathic treatment. Main

> symptoms noted were hot flushes and sweats, tiredness, anxiety, sleeping difficulties, mood swings and headaches. Women referred to homeopathy, were those who either could not take hormone replacement treatment (HRT), or for whom HRT was unsuccessful, or who did not want or who had to come off HRT. The Mean length of homeopathic treatment was 5 months.

I am going to move away from statistics soon, but before I do, I would like to conclude with some information that I am very proud of. The above statistics show that homeopathy's effectiveness proves itself over and over again, at least it does to those who are looking for the truth, rather than those who are prepared to accept a selective biased view of the truth. There is another small and very recent thesis conducted by a graduate student at the University of Johannesburg: *Treatment of Climacteric Symptoms: Case Studies Using Grant Bentley's Method* https://ujdigispace.uj.ac.za/bitstream/handle/10210/9615/Heymans%2c%20SR-2013%20Masters.pdf?sequence=1&isAllowed=y

I stress that the study group was small, but the results are still very impressive. A very précised version is as follows: *The results of the study show a decreasing trend in the Total/Combined MRS. scores, and therefore an increase in the HRQoL of all 9 participants…demonstrated a significant improvement of symptoms after three weeks of homeopathic simillimum treatment, and then a steady amelioration, for the rest of the study period…all 11 symptoms (hot flushes, heart discomfort, insomnia, depressive mood, irritability, anxiety, exhaustion, vaginal dryness, joint and muscular discomfort, and sexual and bladder problems) decreased in severity over the 12-week study period. Homeopathic simillimum treatment appeared to be of benefit in reducing the severity of climacteric symptoms and the Grant Bentley Method showed itself to be a scientific, effective and repeatable method, which enabled the researcher to analyse the case miasmatically and prescribe the appropriate simillimum. This study has contributed to the body of knowledge on the homeopathic treatment of perimenopausal and menopausal symptoms…*

Like all inventors who believe in and have self-validated their work, I was happy to see my work independently evaluated and published. On the surface, it might seem to have nothing to do with the treatment of PANDAS, however the methodology is the same - and the key to success in all of these cases - and I am proud to see others achieve the great results I have been able to realize using this methodology.

If you have already tried and had a positive experience with homeopathy, then you will not care what anyone else says about it; you know it worked for you, or your family, and that is all you will care about. If you are new to homeopathy, or you have never heard of it before, you are probably somewhat confused. 'How can so many scientific studies both prove and disprove homeopathy?' That answer depends on who does the study, as well as who is hand picking the resulting analyses and why. Science is not science when money is involved.

If you are thinking about trying homeopathy for your PANDAS child, but you are concerned about any negative consequences, do not be. When you look at all the negative claims against homeopathy, and listen to the words of the skeptics, none of them ever say that exploring this system means something dangerous might happen; their claim is that nothing will happen at all. The only danger claims you ever read, are from homeopathic opponents trying to warn prospective patients about the risks of coming off or stopping conventional treatments. However, if the only risk you face using homeopathy is the risk that may occur by stopping conventional medication – then do not stop it. Hey presto – problem solved.

15

EXPLAINING HOMEOPATHY

In writing about homeopathy, I am more than aware that I am talking to four different groups.

1. Those who know nothing about homeopathy, but have an interest because someone close to them has PANDAS or PANS.
2. Those who have used and know a little about homeopathy, and have had enough success to keep them exploring.
3. Those who have a PANDAS child and have done a lot of research into homeopathy.
4. Homeopathic practitioners or students who want to know more about PANDAS from an experienced practitioner.

Catering to all these groups is a challenge because it makes this section a balancing act; not putting in too much homeopathic jargon so that newcomers get lost and baffled, and being too basic and boring for readers who already have homeopathic experience.

What I have decided to do is to break this section into two parts. In the first part, I will discuss what homeopathy is, and a little bit about how it works. Then I will discuss the method I have developed, and how it originated from conventional homeopathy in its most classical form, with the addition of a new diagnostic, to aid remedy selection.

What is Homeopathy?

Homeopathy developed from a need to systemize what was essentially at the time, a free for all in medicine. Conventional medicine in the late 1700's to early 1800's was unorganized by today's standards, and very much open to individual interpretation. Ironically, a little like where homeopathy finds itself today. However, I will explain the divergence of homeopathy in part two.

Samuel Hahnemann, the inventor of homeopathy, was a medically trained doctor from Germany, with a gift for logic and observation. Homeopathy is Europe's second oldest alternative medical system after herbalism. If you don't include herbal medicine, as some writers don't, due to the fact that there was little if any formal training in herbal medicine in the 1700's, then homeopathy is Europe's oldest alternative medicine.

Right from its beginning, homeopathy has been embroiled in controversy, but beyond that, it has continually thwarted, annoyed, and amazed conventional medicine and science by surviving at all, when they expected it to die long ago. Not only is homeopathy not dead, despite the huge amounts of energy thrown into killing it, homeopathy is today one of the world's most widespread and used medical systems. Regular medicine expected homeopathy to die because they believed it did not work. Homeopathy is still alive due to patients who have found that it did work and still does work.

The controversy over the efficacy of homeopathy stems not so much from the fact that patients swear that it works, but because it should not work according to science. That of course is also dependent on accepting that science has nothing more to learn because its knowledge is, as of this moment, fool proof and complete. I will leave that with you.

I have discussed about energy in food and how Einstein proved via his $E=MC^2$ work, that there is energy in all things. This energy is inside everything from inorganic substances such as rocks and minerals, to the energy in living beings such as animals, plants, and ourselves.

Einstein's E is the energy that makes nuclear weapons go bang. The question is; is splitting the atom to make matter explode the only way of releasing this energy? If you want to make bombs, the answer is yes. If you want to make a homeopathic remedy the answer is no, it is not the only way. This is where the controversy lies. Hahnemann found a way to release the E from every substance on the planet, so we can put that energy into a bottle and apply it to improve health. Knowing exactly how to use the energy effectively, means studying the topic thoroughly – usually a four-year course - but releasing the energy from substances is at the heart of what homeopathy is. So what is the real controversy here? That E does not exist? Or that homeopathy and not science, developed this method first, and now it cannot be adopted at all without admitting that Hahnemann was right?

The second controversy that shrouds homeopathy is the idea of the similimum. New comers will come across this homeopathic term quickly because the similimum is the basis of the homeopathic system. From this point I am going to write as if you accept that Einstein's E is inside everything and not inside everything except us.

Homeopaths refer to the E inside us as being our Vital Force, but it can also be referred to as life force or vitality. Religious people might refer to it as spirit, while shamans and mystics may refer to this force as our aura or astral body. The Chinese call this force chi, and this energy is what acupuncturists move and generate around the body when they place their needles in specific spots. It is the area that yogis work on to enhance spiritual and physical improvement, and it is why yoga makes people feel so wonderful.

Life force is used in a thousand different ways by a thousand different systems, but all have the one same purpose: to make you feel happy, healthy, and balanced, by generating health and vitality within your constitution. Notice that I said constitution and not just the body, because life force enriches more than our physical form; it is also a major contributor to how we think and how we feel.

Some people claim that homeopathy cannot possibly be true and that it does not work at all. They say that even if Hahnemann did find a way of extracting energy from substances, non-physical or energetic properties cannot influence the physical body. Science and skeptics both make this claim, yet on a day-to-day basis we all know that energy does influence us.

Electricity is about as E as you can get and definitely affects the physical body. There are other examples, such as our thoughts. I discussed earlier, how scientific research has shown that our thoughts can trigger a physical response to such a degree, that just thinking about weight training will fire all the same impulses as doing the training itself. Thoughts are E, because thoughts are not physicals things. And what about emotions? Are we going to say that these E's don't affect the way we physically feel, even though depressed people have far greater rates of heart disease, high blood pressure, diabetes, and stroke, when compared to happy people?

Common sense tells us that energy affects us, both physically and emotionally, every day. Let me give you one natural example of how energy influences physical form.

Pretend that for some reason you were able to live long enough to conduct the following experiment. You place some volatile uranium into a box and then wait a few billion years. Then you open that box, and what is inside? Not uranium, but lead.

So how did this happen? It happened because uranium is an element that gives off energy. That means uranium's energy structure is slowly but consistently changing. This experiment also teaches us that a change in energy will also create a corresponding change in physical form because the two are integrally linked.

The physical form of any being or substance must always match the aura that surrounds and envelopes that being. The two are inseparably linked. Uranium is only physically uranium because it has the aura or energy of uranium. Change that energy pattern and the physical structure also changes.

Human beings as a species, and also as individuals, have their own unique energy patterns, and just like uranium, these energy patterns can be altered too.

Uranium naturally decays (gives off energy), and as a result it also changes form. However, uranium is a non-reactive lump of rock and it takes more time than we can imagine to physically change. But people are not lumps of rock. We are conscious and highly reactive, especially the energetic part of who we are. Our thoughts and emotions are energetic. If our mental and emotional (energy) reactions are strong and consistent enough, then just like the uranium, there will be a change in our physical body. If the change in our energy pattern is negative (emotional stress or an adverse view of ourselves) then there will be a corresponding negative change in our body (chronic disease). If our energy is positive, we will stay strong and healthy relative to our age.

When energy is re-arranged and re-organized towards the positive, which alters or at least halts the negative physical consequences that the negative pattern created, a healthy outcome occurs. This is the basic philosophy behind how an energy medicine like homeopathy works.

Samuel Hahnemann, the founder of homeopathy, discovered that every substance has its own unique energy pattern, just like uranium and lead, but he also found that those different energy patterns will affect us in different ways. For some people, a particular energy pattern will have no effect whatsoever, while for other people that same pattern can be deep and even disturbing. How the energy pattern of a substance affects us depends on – you guessed it – our own energy pattern and how the two interact. This relationship, one energy pattern reacting or resonating to another, is called the similimum. The similimum is an energy so similar to your own, it will interact with you and makes changes to your health in a positive way.

16

TYPES OF HOMEOPATHY

This next section is probably only of interest to homeopaths and parents who have used different types of homeopathy before. I have added this information because I get asked about these topics frequently. Both practitioners and parents see the word 'homeopathy' and immediately think 'this substance is homeopathic'. But there is a big difference between a remedy that is potentized (a substance turned into and called a homeopathic remedy) and a remedy that is given to someone homeopathically. That is, given according to homeopathic rules – matching the *similimum* (your energy) via an analysis of your *totality of symptoms* and your *miasm* (internal defense mechanism). Leaving out those important processes means the 'homeopathic' remedy possibly won't do anything at all. If there is no resonance between patient and remedy, there will be little or no result.

Simplexes and Complexes
Homeopaths can use either simplex prescriptions or complex prescriptions. A simplex is where one remedy is used at a time. A complex is where a number of different remedies are mixed into the one vial. Complexes are usually well known because they are easily purchased in pharmacies and health food shops that sell homeopathic products.

However, the similimum given via a simplex or single remedy has always been the true homeopath's goal. The reason for this is both effectiveness and reproducibility. A mixture or complex may alleviate a condition, but it will be doing so because one or two of the remedies in the complex is suitable to the case. But which one or two? There is the argument 'who cares as long as it's working', but nothing works forever. What will happen when the positive effect stops? How will the practitioner know which two remedies, out of a dozen or more, were the most effective agents, so that in the future they can choose other remedies that might be required, due to their relationship to the remedies that first worked? When using a single remedy, you always know which remedy to repeat and what avenue to take once a patient has a good response.

Acute and Chronic Disease

These two terms are vital for a homeopath to differentiate when deciding how to treat a patient. These terms refer to the classification of the presenting symptoms.

A true acute disease is usually an infectious disease. This means its origins are from something external. This could be an infection from a virus such as the common cold, or it could be a bacterial infection like the streptococcal bacteria so familiar in PANDAS. An acute disease or an acute infection is limited by its time frame. Most acute illnesses will only last a week or two, although there are some exceptions, such as whooping cough which can last much longer.

A chronic disease is different to an acute in two ways. First, it lasts a much longer time; for many it can last a lifetime. Second, a chronic disease does not have a peak of suffering, nor does it taper out and resolve in the end. In fact, exactly the opposite tends to happen. An acute disease can start with some mild discomfort, but then the symptoms go wild for a while, creating havoc in the system and then start to subside. A chronic disease often starts out mildly, but continues to worsen as the years go by. It has no calming of symptoms and it has no resolution at the end. Generally, with a chronic disease, the older you get, the worse your condition becomes.

These two categories are important to this book because they are integral to the way I practice, and different to some methods within homeopathy.

Classical Homeopathy and the HFA Method

I want to discuss the differences between conventional (often referred to as classical) homeopathic treatment and the method by which I practice. I consider myself a classical homeopath (a practitioner who adheres to the original foundations of homeopathy) but I have added a new diagnostic (facial analysis) and have further divided classification of disease.

Following on from my previous discussion on disease classification, in standard classical homeopathy, there are only the two classifications: acute and chronic. Both, according to traditional Hahnemannian thinking, result from an infection. My point of difference is that there should be a third classification related to chronic disease and that is the classification of a non-infectious chronic disease. Diseases like tuberculosis are chronic by definition, but so too are diseases such as arthritis or cancer. The difference is that arthritis and cancer have no single infectious cause, whereas tuberculosis or other chronic infectious diseases such as AIDS do.

This point of difference is huge. It may seem like a small point of difference, but I assure you it is anything but that, and in some ways it is why my practice is so successful.

Let me get specific and make PANDAS the center of what I am talking about. PANDAS is an acute disease - right or wrong? The answer is that PANDAS is a chronic disease that has acute exacerbations. This means a PANDAS child can have acute flare ups of their symptoms because of an infection like strep, but overall PANDAS is a chronic disease, because patients have a tendency to flare via a variety of circumstances.

PANDAS kids can go into a flare when a cold virus hits the household. But PANDAS kids can also flare if they eat sugar, drink red cordial, or eat wheat too often. PANDAS kids can flare if they lose too much sleep, and they can flare if they are anxious, worried, or exhausted. But exhaustion is not an infection. The reason this theory (the non-infection chronic disease theory) is important, is because understanding the relationship between PANDAS and non-infectious chronic disease is the crux of success in my clinical practice.

Classical homeopathy is an important way of practicing homeopathy that is mainly focused on chronic disease. Its philosophy is simple. The whole constitution – mind, emotions, and body – are affected during the chronic disease, so the whole constitution needs to be examined in order to find the right single or simplex remedy. There are no complex constitutional remedies. For this reason, and that a practitioner can manage a case more effectively when single remedies are given, one at a time, I am a strong supporter of this aspect of classical homeopathy.

Miasms
There is another important area with homeopathy that is widely discussed but not used very much in the clinical setting. If you know even a little about homeopathy, you will have come across the term miasm.

A miasm is a term used since the early 1800's, within homeopathy, to describe a genetically inherited disease. The concept was written about extensively, to help make clear where chronic disease came from. It is ironic for me that this topic – miasms - which led me to research facial analysis and to develop Homeopathic Facial Analysis (HFA), should still cause so much confusion within the homeopathic world. Homeopaths either ignore the miasm or they try to remove it. I have come to clearly understand that the miasm is the defense mechanism of the patient. An important part of the patient – not to be ignored, or to be removed. It is the signpost to understanding how that patient faces their own world and their own pattern of illness. It is the signpost to finding the deepest acting remedies that will help the patient to find balance within their own chronic condition.

Samuel Hahnemann (the founder of homeopathy who lived from 1755 till 1843) spent 12 years thinking about, and observing through clinical practice, an underlying concept of chronic disease. He saw that chronic disease kept returning when certain conditions were in place. Hahnemann still hoped the underlying factor could be removed, but my experience has shown me that chronic illness can only be managed and not annihilated. Because our chronic disease is, in essence, how we respond to stress. The trick is to manage both the stress and the response.

In my opinion, the reason why Hahnemann was so rigid about the existence of the miasm, was because he had no other way of conceptualizing and explaining how a patient with a chronic disease improved. He knew that patients suffering from an acute disease got better because the remedy in some way 'pushed out' the invading bacteria or virus. If a patient with a chronic disease was getting better under a remedy, then something must have been pushed out, hence there must have been a pre-existing virus or bacteria in the first place.

This way of thinking implies that energy only works in one way. If you go back to basic chemistry, you will remember that there are always as many neutrons in a nucleus as there are protons in an element, unless it is an isotope. The reason there are neutrons, is for them to act as a buffer to the protons. It is the only way the universe can build on itself. Protons have a positive charge, and just like the two same poles of a magnet, two positive charges will repel each other. They need a neutron between them to neutralize the charge.

Hahnemann mentions the action of magnets in his writings, so it is clear he understood this analogy when trying to explain the action of homeopathy. It is important to know that Hahnemann firstly invented and applied homeopathy, then wrote about these outcomes and finally tried to explain homeopathy's action. For many practitioners, these two areas have become confused – the action of homeopathy, and the explanation of homeopathy. But the action of magnets is important, because it shows us how acute disease responds to the action of remedies – through positive to positive repulsion.

But when you apply the logic of repelling a disease from the body in regard to chronic disease, it doesn't fit what is actually happening. I thought about this long and hard before it dawned on me. Energy does not perform a single function. Energy not only repels, energy also replenishes. Energy is not one sided, it is multifaceted. Energy invigorates and empowers, it is so much more than just a repelling force.

Understanding that energy replenishes is why the remedies I choose work at such a deep level with my PANDAS patients. They rebuild and repair the body; they don't repel a genetic virus. And this is why your PANDAS child has flares whenever they become tired. This is why your PANDAS child has flares if they become overly excited. This is why your PANDAS child has flares when they are sick, when they have eaten the wrong foods, or when they are stressed and tired from school, cutting a new tooth, or going through a growth spurt. In homeopathic language, PANDAS is an energy disease, not just a bacterial one.

Yes, it is true that strep can push these kids over the edge, but so too can a dozen other infections. The key to understanding how to treat and manage a PANDAS child is to know about their energetic homeostasis.

This change in how to view a PANDAS patient might seem simple enough, but seeing their illness in this way has a huge ramification in practice. Some of the following news will be what you as a parent want to hear, some of it will not. What you want hear is that complete cure is right around the corner and often after the first dose. Even though single doses rarely bring about deep change, there is real lasting genuine help available. You just have to swap the idea of a permanent cure, to an effective management and treatment strategy.

Management is the key to PANDAS because PANDAS is an energy disease and energy needs to be managed – it cannot be pushed out or eradicated. When parents know their child has an energy disease, it also means that they don't have to have to panic each time their child experiences a flare. It does not mean that the treatment has failed and there are no further options if their child has some regression. It simply means they need to understand that right at this time, there is more of their PANDAS child's energy going out than coming in. Something, and it could be anything - an acute illness, poor diet, stress, physical fatigue - something is upsetting their energy balance. The job of the homeopathic remedy is to put this imbalance back into balance.

So this is why homeopathy is such an important part of my treatment plan for PANDAS and why I stress it forms the foundation of treatment with every case of PANDAS. As a naturopath, I am trained to use any number of other modalities including diet. But PANDAS is an energy disturbance and that means the type of treatment I use must be equally as energetic. Homeopathy is energy with a capital E.

Case 7
Cody – male aged 13 years
Cody had been diagnosed with PANDAS and PANS, as well as Lyme disease and the typical co-infections of Bartonella and Babesia. Although the diagnosis had been recent, the typical PANDAS behaviors, if typical is the right word to describe something that varies so much, had been present for many years.

Cody's main complaints included oppositional defiance, video game addiction (although this is hardly limited to PANDAS), sleeping problems, multiple food allergies, fears, anxiety, intrusive thoughts, bedwetting, and tics, both vocal and physical. His vocal tics commonly included the repeating under his breath of any answer he gave to a question, a convulsive hand movement that Cody has learned to disguise by pretending to scratch an itch, and an eye rolling tic that he could not disguise and which led him to being teased at school.

None of these tics or behaviors had developed since the diagnosis of PANDAS, nor had they been in anyway alleviated by the repeated doses of Augmentin he had been prescribed. I have noted (in my clinic) that around half of all my PANDAS patients don't respond to repeated antibiotic treatment.

Cody was intellectually normal with good social skills. He could understand subtext and he could grasp subtlety, metaphor, and irony. PANDAS is a disturbance that can affect all sorts of kids. A child can have PANDAS and yet in every other way be intellectually and socially normal, or they may have autism and PANDAS, which is a different and infinitely more complex issue.

The more a condition fluctuates in its presentation, the greater the chance I have of bringing that patient back into balance. If a PANDAS child has good days and bad days, then that PANDAS child has a far greater chance of being stabilized and advancing more quickly, than a child who has little if any mental or emotional fluctuations in behavior.

For example, if a child is severely autistic or has Down's syndrome, as well as symptoms of PANDAS that flare when they are ill, during a full moon, or when they eat dairy, then the chances of being able to positively influence the PANDAS symptoms is high, simply because their condition responds to energy changes. However, the chances of being able to do anything remarkable with severe autism or Down's syndrome separate from the PANDAS, is far less likely because these conditions do not fluctuate in accordance to personal energy. This does not mean that treatment won't help improve severely autistic or Down's syndrome children generally. I have seen many kids in these two groups physically improve and sometimes even make steps forward intellectually. They might start eating with a spoon instead of with their hands, or pat the dog once or twice whereas before they seemed unaware that it even existed. These steps forward are significant but they are not remarkable.

On the other hand, I have seen many remarkable steps forward when it comes to the treatment of what I will call uncomplicated PANDAS.

Cody presented with uncomplicated PANDAS. Like a lot of PANDAS kids, he had always been quirky, or as his mother said, 'he has always had his little ways.' But ways and quirkiness are just the shades of complexity in being human. You can't have individuality without difference. What makes us skilled, distinctive, or sometimes even attractive, is our difference, not our sameness.

One of Cody's individual ways was an unquenchable interest in all things spiritual. He loved chants and had memorized long medieval prayers. He adored sermons and loved the idea of angels, but at the same time he was also obsessed by the thought of demons, and he was tormented by the prospect of hell. When Cody was in a flare, every negative thought he had was the devil tempting him, and because he had evil thoughts, it meant the devil was winning and he was failing.

During our Skype consultation, he asked me questions about homeopathy and how the concept of energy changed the idea of life as we understand it. Profound questions that I wouldn't expect from most adults, let alone a thirteen-year-old boy. In some ways, Cody was born into the wrong time. Five hundred years ago he would have had his own following and been revered as a holy man. But this consultation took place in 2014, so Cody was considered an oddball and ill.

It took me a few attempts before finding a remedy that finally did something positive. Even then, it took some remedy changes to find one that worked the deepest for him, but when I did find the right group of remedies, everything changed for Cody.

The first symptom to subside was his eye-rolling tic and for this he was very grateful. Despite the schools no bullying policy, he was still teased, but just in a subtler way. However, after only a few months of treatment, his facial tics were almost gone. Cody's vocal tic was also greatly diminished within the first few months of treatment, but still evident if he got very tired or felt very stressed.

The other physical change that occurred along with the alleviation and disappearance of the tics was his bedwetting. When I first met Cody he was having a bedwetting episode at least four times a week, and when it did occur, it was copious. At the same time as his eye-rolling tic started decreasing, so too did his bedwetting, something for which I think his mother was even more happy about than Cody himself.

A month after the eye-rolling tic had reached a level that would be considered gone, Cody's fears and intrusive thoughts regarding the supernatural world had also decreased significantly, and by significantly, it was about a subjective ninety percent or more decrease, to a point where these negative thoughts were virtually imperceptible. His positive interest in the spiritual world remained just as high, which I find interesting, as it goes to show that as Cody became more and more balanced in himself, his interests and passions stayed the same while the expression and intensity of what was tormenting him changed. This shows that inside us there are two states of being. In Cody's case, there was his passion for spiritual knowledge which did not change after treatment because it is part of his personality, and there was his out of balanced tormented state, which was clearly a manifestation linked directly to his state of internal stress. This second state is not part of Cody's personality, but a visible projection of his inward turmoil.

I have observed these dual states in many patients, and as with Cody, the negative state that is triggered by stress took a back place, because the action of the remedy balanced out his energetic state. (I have written more about the two states of personality that exist in us all, in my book, *Soul and Survival*)

Over the next few months, Cody's scratching tic disappeared and so too, as is often the case during treatment, his hypersensitivity to certain foods. As already discussed, this did not mean that Cody could eat foods like sugar everyday with impunity, but it did mean that he could enjoy a treat every now and then without the household suffering.

The only times Cody's PANDAS reoccurs now is right before he gets sick with a cold or whatever other virus might be going around, or if he gets very nervous with anticipation before a test. Other than that he is a happy healthy functioning kid, with a good social life and a very inquisitive mind.

For Homeopaths
The following rubrics were selected for Cody's repertorisation –

> MIND; ANXIETY; salvation, about (37)
> MIND; RELIGIOUS affections (72)
> EYE; MOVEMENT; eyeballs; convulsive, spasmodic (24)
> BLADDER; URINATION; involuntary; night, incontinence in bed (143)
> MIND; FEAR; ghosts, of (41)

I included two rubrics in this repertorisation that are a little more of a symbolic extrapolation than what Cody actually said. At the same time, I believe these rubrics are in keeping with the general essence of what he said. For example, his fear of the devil and of going to hell have been represented by the rubrics – 'Anxiety; salvation' and 'Fear; ghosts.' Literal rubrics regarding hell and the devil were too small for me to use, while 'salvation' has the same connotation, but more remedies in the rubric. His fear of the devil and demons has been symbolized by the bigger remedy rubric of 'Fear; ghosts.'

As stated, my first remedy attempts did not yield anything positive, mainly because I had his facial analysis wrong. Not because of the quality of the photos, but because his face was particularly hard to read. As with anything in life, some people and procedures are straight forward and some are not.

After re-analyzing Cody's facial features I considered that he belonged to the yellow group (psora). This means Cody deals with stress and disease by throwing anything harmful outward. As a result, he must have a constitutional remedy that shares that same outward motion.

The first outward remedy of choice was Sulphur. This was chosen because it repertorised up the highest. Patients and other homeopaths sometimes ask why I choose remedies that don't seem to fit the patient? I reply that all of my remedies fit the patient and I have the repertorisation to prove it. What they are referring to of course is profiling a patient to the stereotype of the remedy – the 'Sulphur type' or the 'Lycopodium type,' but I don't subscribe to typecasting. What am I trying to fix? The patient's condition. Has my repertorisation accurately included the main symptoms of the patient's condition? Yes. Are those accurately portrayed symptoms (rubrics), found within the sphere of the remedy? Yes. Then I have a matched the patient to the remedy.

While Sulphur alleviated the symptoms a little bit, and so too did Pulsatilla, it was Lycopodium that did all the work and took Cody from being a PANDAS kid, to a normal kid with some unusual interests. Lycopodium was given in 30C daily.

17

A NEW WAY TO LOOK AT HOMEOPATHY

What I want to do now is highlight some of the differences between the way I practice, compared to some concepts in classical homeopathy. If homeopathy is completely new to you, this might seem insignificant, but for practitioners it is important to know when a result is good and how to manage a case in the longer term.

I wrote before about swapping the term management for cure. Classical homeopathy places a lot of emphasis on curing disease, whatever that disease many be. Would anyone in any kind of practice think that Cody's outcome was not a success? No, of course not. Most practitioners, regardless of their modality, would be over the moon to achieve a result like this, just as I was. Cody can now go weeks, or months, with hardly any PANDAS symptoms at all. However, if he gets run down or he gets a cold, he will often flare again. But typically nowhere near to the same degree as before. He uses the remedy through the period of the cold, and then after the cold is over, his PANDAS symptoms die down again. This pattern of reoccurrence means by definition, that Cody has not been cured.

Even though I said earlier that the bad news is I don't believe in absolute and permanent cure for chronic disease, Cody is a great example of what effective homeopathic management can do. He is ninety-nine percent better, ninety-five percent of the time, and anyone that is not happy with that type of outcome is either a non-practicing homeopathic philosopher who has never learned the difference between theory and real practice, or someone who has never had to deal with PANDAS. Cody's mum isn't complaining and neither am I.

The next area of difference between classical homeopathy and the way I practice, is replacing the notion that every symptom has an infectious origin, to the idea that every symptom is an outward expression of how balanced a patient's system is at any given point.

What we see with Cody, is that every time he gets nervous before a test, or his body is fighting a cold, he gets a mild to moderate return of his old PANDAS symptoms. It can also happen if he eats too much sugar. Now if we are going to stick with the infectious model of classical homeopathy, we also have to say that it's sheer bad luck that every time Cody eats sugar or is about to sit an exam he also gets re-infected with the same virus that caused his original PANDAS. It is too incredulous to believe that a germ is causing every flare, when through observation, it becomes obvious that different types of stress – from bacterial, to environmental, to dietary, to emotional – can be the trigger. And most importantly, even though every patient should try to avoid triggers, the main inroad a natural approach and a well-chosen homeopathic remedy can achieve, is to moderate the patient's response to a level where the patient can manage their own environment and their own personal state effectively.

Homeopathy has an interesting place in the world. Both medical and mystical, it attracts both scientists and those who follow any rule a homeopathic leader puts forward. Some treat homeopathy as if it's a religion that cannot be changed. These fundamentalists are often very vocal and adamant certain rules must be followed. I have spoken to many of them and sadly many don't practice even though they are fascinated by homeopathy. Outside of the time I put aside for writing, I am in full time practice, I always have been, and that means I have certain practical realities that supersede any academic fantasy. My practical reality is getting patients better and I never get sick of hearing how someone feels better because of what I have been able to do for them. I've been getting a buzz from that for more than two decades and I still love it.

Back to the story of my homeopathic difference. About fifteen years ago now, I had to question myself; 'Why am I not getting the consistent results I want?' Why are too many of my patients not responding?' I knew the rules of classical homeopathy, I knew what all the old masters and experts said to do. I ought to, I had been teaching this information at college level for ten years, so I knew the difference between rules and the results that come from following those rules. I knew which rules were rules and which rules should be treated as guidelines. I knew which rules were laws of nature and therefore must be followed, and which rules were really personal opinions masquerading as rules. If you are a homeopath or a serious student, I lay all of this information out in another book I wrote, *How Aphorism 27 Changed the World*.

There I was nearly twenty years ago, observing what I saw in the clinic, what was written by the old masters including Hahnemann himself, and reading about, and testing, many of the new ideas being presented by other homeopaths. I was not alone. There were a number of homeopaths trying to perfect the way they used homeopathy clinically, and also trying to understand how it worked. I decided to throw every opinion and every foundation, except the similimum, which is the basic foundation of homeopathy, out the window and I started again. From that basis, I kept only what I knew clinically worked and what was reproducible, and then I built my own personal philosophy around those aspects, so I could understand why they were working.

I was careful to keep the basic foundations of homeopathy. The law of similars, the concept of totality, and the single well-chosen remedy. I knew that Hahnemann's miasm theory was important, yet it was being used in a number of different ways or else completely ignored. I knew that two well respected homeopaths (Allen and Roberts), had made minor references to facial structure and Hahnemann's miasm model, but had not taken these ideas any further.

Out of both curiosity and a desire to understand why Hahnemann put so much emphasis on the concept of a miasm as part of his own clinical practice, I began my own research project. Within five years I was using the face as a key diagnostic to every patient's internal defense system. And my results became deeper, stronger, and most importantly, consistent. I was thrilled and so were my patients. I began to share my new concept which became known as Homeopathic Facial Analysis (HFA), and to date, I am proud to say that this model is practiced by homeopaths in 25 countries and is starting to be taught in homeopathic schools, including the Johannesburg University previously mentioned.

I had no idea my curiosity would take me on this pathway. I love getting feedback from other practitioners and students, but my main focus is still within the clinic where it all began. My success with PANDAS is due solely to the information I get from the face, along with the use of the classical concepts of totality and the single remedy. My dosing has changed dramatically, but that is in part due to my complete understanding of the energetic action of homeopathic remedies.

18

E = ENERGY

I want you now to cast your mind back to when I was talking about energy working in more than the one (repellent) way. Remember how I said that energy replenishes as well?

Think of what was happening inside Cody. If you have any biology experience, think of energy as something within us that exists within upper and lower levels, like blood sugar or blood gases. If our blood sugar goes too far above its homeostatic range, then symptoms of hyperglycemia are produced. If it goes too far under then symptoms of hypoglycemia are produced.

Our energy levels have their own homeostatic range and PANDAS symptoms will return if those levels go too hyper or too hypo. If Cody loses too much sleep, his symptoms will return because his energy has gone into the hypo range. If he gets stressed before a test, or he eats too much sugar, he will go into the hyper range and again his PANDAS symptoms will return. To a complete materialist who doesn't believe in energy, this concept will be regarded as unprovable. But to a PANDAS parent who has been observing their child, this concept explains a lot. That's why I call PANDAS an energy disease or an energy disturbance, and why homeopathy is such an important part of the treatment process.

My next digression from classical homeopathy is with the single dose. Hahnemann talked of giving one dose and then to wait for a response, until he developed a regime of repeating the dose with a different potency scale (the LM's). But giving single doses and waiting won't do when it comes to PANDAS. PANDAS kids are highly reactive because their energy levels are unstable, so they need a constant input of usable energy to keep them balanced. The more hyper, angry, or anxious, the more consistently the remedy needs to be applied.

Another difference, and this has been huge and the whole basis of my system, is in how I find the right remedy. There are thousands, maybe tens of thousands of homeopathic remedies to choose from. How do you find the one, two, or three, that are going to stabilize your child? Remember when I spoke about the uranium turning into lead? You were probably thinking, 'What on earth is this guy going on about?' Maybe you still do? I hope not. Anyway, I spoke about how energy patterns relate specifically to the physical form they are connected to. When energy is used for health it must be specific. But energy is something you can't see, so how do you know which remedies will have a similar energy to the patient before giving it to them?

That very question took me years to figure out, but the bottom line is, there is a way. The energy of uranium creates a different physical structure to lead. Change the energy and you change the form. But what if there was a way to reverse that equation so you could know the energy by analyzing the form? After all, we may not be able to see energy, but we can certainly see and evaluate physical form. After years of what was at times excruciating and painstaking detail, in the end I did figure out a way by analyzing the most expressive and most unique physical aspect of ourselves – the face.

Now when I think about it, trying to assess physical structure so I could understand the individual energy that created that structure is obvious. And what other feature could be used? It had to be our face. We can be waiting for a friend at a show or a sporting event. Hundreds, maybe thousands of people walk past us while we're waiting. Many of these people are the same height, many more will share the same eye color, and at least half will be the same gender, but you will recognise your friend the moment you see them, because nothing, apart from fingerprints, is more individually distinctive than our face. Hence the name, Homeopathic Facial Analysis, or HFA.

Every patient has their photograph taken, or more precisely, has numerous photographs taken of their face. It's a bit like going to jail, except that I ask you to smile. If you are seeing me via Skype, then each patient gets a set of instructions on how to take the photos. Either way, a facial analysis is done, measuring sizes and angles, symmetry and shape. (HFA has nothing whatsoever to do with how you look or your general appearance or expressions, that is not what is being assessed).

This process means I can narrow down dramatically the type of remedy I am looking for. It doesn't mean I will find the best remedy first go out of the thousands of available remedies, but it doesn't mean I won't find it first go either. Clinical statistics from feedback from a number of clinics using the HFA process, show that 80% of patients received some degree of improvement within the first four remedies, with 50% of those 80% claiming their improvement to be significant. Using the face to group patients and to find remedies that bring about deep change, makes a big difference.

19

ERRONEOUS IDEAS IN HOMEOPATHY

There are a number of ideas within homeopathy that I don't subscribe to. Like many other homeopaths, I was taught these ideas and I am fully aware where they came from and why. As I began to work more with only the basic principles of homeopathy – the totality of symptoms and the miasm – and my idea of the miasm changed from a disease model to a defense system model, I reviewed and tested some of these ideas and found them lacking.

Layers of Treatment
If you're a new comer and you have no idea what I'm talking about, trust me you are better off. As for the rest of us, I spend more time talking about this damnable subject than any other topic. This 'layers' idea is an extension of the 'everything comes down to an acquired disease' theory, because a layer is meant to be a past disease that needs to be removed. According to the theory, you haven't just inherited one layer of illness, but each generation, before and including your own, has added more and more disease ridden sediment layers to your now over-burdened system. Only once these hurdles have been overcome, will the body finally begin to be free and healthy again. The problem is, these layers that homeopaths talk about theoretically

date back to Adam, literally if you are a fundamentalist Christian, and figuratively if you're not.

The way I see it, I did not remove any layers from Cody, or if I did, it was by sheer accident and unbeknown to me. However, if I had inadvertently removed the layer that was causing Cody's PANDAS, then why did that layer return the moment he got stressed? I'm sure you could come up with some hypothetical reason to keep the whole argument going, but to me the energy conclusion is obvious, and the more I have learned how to use the energy model, the more successful as a practitioner I have become.

To me, what's right is what works. So in answer to the question about homeopathic protocols to remove layers? All I can say is what I've already said. PANDAS is an energetic disturbance; it is not something you catch. The fact that it can be triggered by a strep infection, does not mean it is a strep infection. If it was, antibiotics would have more than a short term affect.

Anti-doting
This topic concerns other treatments and the anti-doting or prevention of the action of remedies. Classical homeopathy has two main theoretical anti-doting hurdles – neither of which I subscribe to. The first is in regard to conventional medicines and the second involves other allied antidotes. As part of classical theory, there is an idea that any conventional medicine, from steroids to antibiotics, to anti-inflammatories and everything in between, will not just disrupt but halt and antidote any homeopathic given at the same time.

Supposedly, homeopathy and conventional medicine cannot be used at the same time. Other antidotes to homeopathic remedies, that supposedly cannot be taken or used at the same time, include toothpaste, some deodorants, and coffee, just to name a few.

Based on nearly a quarter of a century of continuous clinical practice, my opinion on anti-doting is that it is rubbish. The right remedy continues to act as long as it resonates to the patient and their symptoms. The right remedy creates a positive flow and once started, it is difficult to stop – not that anyone would want that outcome.

Conventional Medicine
As a parent of a PANDAS child I can tell you directly that you do not have to choose between a doctor or a homeopath, as the two can work perfectly well together even if your doctor disagrees.

I have treated many PANDAS kids and adult patients who take conventional medications as required or even on a daily basis. The only request I have is that a patient does not start any additional medicines at the same time as they start taking their remedy, but as for the medications they are already on, I suggest they keep taking them until they are healthy enough not to need them anymore. I have never taken any patient off a prescription medication. That is between the patient and their doctor. It is not my role to challenge the place of conventional medicine, it is my role to get patients' back to better health, and there is no better reason to give up medicine than good health.

If you come to see me as a patient and you are already on medication, you are still going to tell me about symptoms X, Y and Z, because that's what you have come to me for. I will still be able to tell whether my remedies are working by assessing the progress of X, Y and Z. Taking existing medication does not hinder my ability to assess a case, and it certainly does not antidote any of the homeopathic remedies.

So if strong medications don't inhibit remedies, then coffee and toothpaste have no chance of affecting them. I don't know how or why this idea has become such an accepted truth, but it is nonsense. If a remedy wasn't strong enough to cut through toothpaste, what hope would it have of unraveling PANDAS?

Mixing Alternative Treatments
The only real inhibiting factor, and this is a very touchy subject that needs to be approached with sensitivity, are parents who panic and

make a full time job out of searching for PANDAS treatments. I understand the desperation, and I understand the pain when seeing their child experience these awful symptoms. I understand the fear they experience, and the soul tearing sympathy created by seeing their child battle with their own mind. Seeing their own child delusional or paranoid can make a parent fall to their knees, BUT coming up with extra solutions and treatments before the first remedy has even been given a chance to work often slows down and hinders the progress of treatment.

Managing PANDAS, as every PANDAS parent knows, is a delicate and very difficult path. Treating PANDAS is no road for the blind, it requires skill and experience and a touch of finesse. These kids, as we already know, are super sensitive and hyper reactive. You cannot keep throwing every idea you have, down their throat the moment you have it, in the hope that one of these ideas will hit the spot. Hyper-reactive means your PANDAS child needs less complexity in their day to day management, not more. Too many treatments will only confuse their system and throw it into further disarray.

20

SUPPORTIVE PARENTS

Homeopathy can be a miracle, but it is not always enough on its own. Stabilizing a PANDAS child is a joint effort between myself and the primary care giver, usually the mother. I rely on her observations and her analysis just as much as my own. She is an active participant in this process and my job is infinitely harder if she is not involved. I might be the one that tells her what she needs to look out for and why, but she is the one who is doing the observing. I am not the one who is going to be cooking for her PANDAS child, and I am not the one patiently listening to her child when they are upset and distressed. I just hear the details after the fact, during the next consultation. It is the mother or sometimes the father who provides me with the information I need, so that together we can work out what needs to be done.

PANDAS is a condition that doesn't have to be accepted. It is a condition that can be calmed, and it can be effectively managed. And not just for the short term, but consistently. As a large and ever growing number of socially accepted kids, balanced kids, tic free kids, baseball playing kids, unrestricted diet kids, sleeping in their own room kids, un-tormented free thinking kids, and most important of all, happy kids, will testify.

FIND OUT MORE

If you want to learn more about HFA homeopathy please see the Victorian College of Classical Homeopathy website www.vcch.org. This site highlights cases, online training, consultation information, and general information about the development of HFA. I can be contacted through this site via the college office. I welcome queries, feedback, and your interest, especially for your PANDAS child.

AUTHOR BIOGRAPHY

Grant Bentley
ND Dip Hom Grad Dip Psych. Th reg AROH, ATMS
Grant Bentley is from Melbourne, Australia and has been working and studying in various fields of natural therapies since 1987. Grant is a qualified Homeopath and Naturopath and has studied Clinical Hypnosis and has a Post Graduate Diploma in Eriksonian Psychotherapy.

Grant has been in clinical practice for over 25 years. Treating children with PANDAS is a major part of his clinical focus and he is now regarded as a world expert and the leading authority in the homeopathic treatment of this condition.

In the 1990's Grant became the principal of the Victorian College of Classical Homeopathy; a college known for its high academic standards in classical homeopathic philosophy together with a practical results based clinic. In the late 1990's Grant began a research project on facial structure and miasms. This project became a new homeopathic methodology known as Homeopathic Facial Analysis (HFA). Since its development HFA has been taught to both undergraduate and postgraduate students around the world. To date, practitioners in more than 25 countries use HFA.

At its core, HFA is a method that allows a homeopathic practitioner to select remedies that work in harmony with a patient's system in order to bring it into balance more quickly than contemporary homeopathic treatment. Trials into HFA have been conducted in the private clinics of Grant Bentley as well as a number of Melbourne based VCCH graduates. Trials were also undertaken at the Orwil St Community House clinic (Frankston). Consistent results across numerous chronic diseases including depression, anxiety, asthma, arthritis, migraines, IBS, psoriasis, allergies, eating disorders, behavioral disorders, and weakened immune systems were experienced. The treatment of PANDAS has shown just as much success.

Grant is the author of four previous books: *Appearance and Circumstance (2003), Homœopathic Facial Analysis* (2006). These two books have been combined and published for Asia renamed *Facial Analysis and Homeopathy* (BJain 2011). His other books include: *Soul & Survival* (2008) and *How Aphorism 27 Changed The World* (2012). *Appearance and Circumstance* and *Homœopathic Facial Analysis* have been translated into Russian, German, Spanish and Bulgarian. *Soul & Survival* has been translated into Russian and German. Grant has lectured in Australia, New Zealand, the Middle East, India, USA, Canada, and Europe.

Further information about Grant Bentley's research and his books can be found on these websites

- Victorian College of Classical Homeopathy website www.vcch.org (Miasm research, What is HFA?, HFA training)

GRANT BENTLEY

Contact details
Grant Bentley
PO Box 804
Mt Eliza, Victoria
Australia 3930

admin@vcch.org

Made in the USA
Coppell, TX
11 March 2023

14147318R00085